Avoiding Opioid Abuse
While Managing Pain

**by Lynn R. Webster, MD
and Beth Dove**

Foreword by Steven D. Passik, PhD,
Associate Attending Psychologist,
Memorial Sloan Kettering Cancer Center
Associate Professor of Psychiatry,
Weill College of Cornell Medical Center

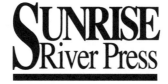

Library of Congress Cataloging-in-Publication Data

Webster, Lynn R.
    Avoiding opioid abuse while managing pain : a guide for practitioners / by Lynn R. Webster and Beth Dove.
        p. ; cm.
    Includes bibliographical references.
    ISBN 978-0-9624814-8-2
    1. Opioids--Therapeutic use. 2. Chronic pain--Chemotherapy--Complications. 3. Opiod abuse--Treatment. 4. Opioids--Side effects. I. Dove, Beth. II. Title.
    [DNLM: 1. Opioid-Related Disorders--prevention & control. 2. Analgesics, Opioid--adverse effects. 3. Analgesics, Opioid--therapeutic use. 4. Pain--drug therapy. 5. Risk Factors. WM 284 W381a 2007]

RC483.5.O64W43 2007
615'.7822--dc22
                        2007015844

ISBN-13 978-0-9624814-8-2

39966 Grand Avenue
North Branch, MN 55056 USA
(651) 277-1400 or (800) 895-4585

TABLE OF CONTENTS

ABOUT THE AUTHORS

Lynn Webster

Lynn Webster, MD, lectures widely on the subject of preventing opioid abuse and criminal diversion in chronic pain patients. Dr. Webster is board certified in anesthesiology and pain management and is certified in addiction medicine. In his private practice, he treats chronic pain patients, many of whom have complex diagnoses. He also treats opioid-addicted patients.

Dr. Webster is medical director of Lifetree Clinical Research and Pain Clinic in Salt Lake City, Utah. His clinical research interests include pain and pain mechanisms, substance abuse and addiction, and the relationship between sleep and pain. A primary focus is the development of innovative analgesic agents that resist abuse. His research has led to the publication of numerous scientific abstracts, articles and textbook chapters, including a contribution to the upcoming first Textbook of Pain and Chemical Dependency (Oxford University Press). He has authored or coauthored articles in journals that include *Pain Medicine*, the *Clinical Journal of Pain, Practical Pain Management,* the *Journal of Opioid Management* and the *American Journal of Therapeutics.*

Dr. Webster earned his doctorate of medicine from the University of Nebraska Medical Center and completed his residency and fellowship with the University of Utah, Department of Anesthesiology and Division of Artificial Organs. He founded the Utah chapter of the American Academy of Pain Medicine. In 2006, Dr Webster began a campaign called Zero Unintentional Deaths (www.zerodeaths.org) to educate healthcare professionals, patients, and communities about the need to increase safety when prescribing or consuming prescription opioids. He established the nonprofit organization LifeSource (www.lsource.org) to raise funds for education and research. This book is part of that campaign to educate healthcare professionals.

Beth Dove

Medical writer and researcher Beth Dove has focused for the past several years on investigating and publishing the facts behind prescription opioid abuse and undertreated pain. She works full time with Dr. Webster. Her technical writing has appeared in *Pain Medicine*, the *Journal of Opioid Management, Practical Pain Management* and many other publications and textbook chapters. She writes educational materials in support of the Zero Unintentional Deaths campaign (www.zerodeaths.org), which is dedicated to ensuring that prescription opioids are safely prescribed and consumed. A former Associated Press and newspaper reporter, she lives with her husband in Salt Lake City, Utah.

FOREWORD

How badly does the field of pain management need books like this one? So badly, in fact, that I am personally editing a textbook on pain and chemical dependency even as I write this foreword. The fields of pain management and chemical dependency desperately need unification both at the 30,000-foot level of theory, hypothesized mechanisms, etc., and also on the ground, in the clinic, where the rubber meets the road. My book (to which Dr. Webster is also a contributor) is a textbook – it provides the 30,000-foot view; this work brings it all together for the practitioner, on the ground, in the clinic, taking care of the complex people in this world with chronic pain. This book provides the know-how to do it safely, avoiding contributing to drug abuse and diversion. Very few people in the country – no, the world - could have written this book. Few have the requisite training, knowledge, intellectual curiosity, tolerance for ambiguity and the passion needed to undertake a work such as this. Dr. Webster is such a person, and here he and his colleague Beth Dove have united to give the data, the clinical experience, and the practical knowledge needed to do it the way they do it - expertly, humanely, safely, and effectively.

When Russell K. Portenoy, MD, Chairman of Pain Medicine and Palluative Care, Beth Israel Hospital, New York, NY, and Kathleen Foley, MD, Director, Soros Foundation Project on Death in America, first urged the pain field to take a new look at opioids in non-cancer pain, they were not simply advocating for an "opening of the flood gates" with regard to prescribing and clinical practice. Instead, they observed that if tertiary care cancer patients exhibit favorable outcomes on opioids (meaningful analgesia, improvements in psychosocial function, manageable side effects, and the absence of addiction), then it stood to reason that *subsets* of the vast and heterogeneous population of people with non-cancer pain could also potentially derive such benefits. It was up to practitioners and scientists to conduct the n of 1 or n of 1001 trials to find out how best to bring about such outcomes in non-cancer pain patients. They called for a medical, scientific, and healthcare-based discussion of this issue, backed up by data and clinical experience, as opposed to the more traditionally legal and ethical debates that had dominated to that point. The need then, as it is now, was to replace rhetoric and opinion with science, experience, knowledge, and reason.

But in our aging society with a growing problem of chronic pain, an abysmal track record of undertreatment, and, as John Bonica, MD, called it, "apathetic therapeutic inactivity," the clinical practice took off faster than clinical trials data could accrue. Rhetoric was used in place of science, and in their zeal to do good, the pain management community seemed to forget that all pain management goes on against the backdrop provided by our substance-abusing society (which goes as we know, far beyond opioids, to nicotine, cannabis, alcohol, and other licit and illicit drugs). The result was a perfect storm: rhetoric, increased prescribing, the availability of new opioids and other agents, and the failure to teach about addiction. In the end, we now have the concomitant and growing problem of prescription drug abuse.

The need for bridging pain and chemical dependency includes the empirical, clinical, and didactic domains. This work addresses primarily the rugged terrain of the clinical treatment of pain with opioids. For the good of our patients and their communities, all prescribers of controlled substances need to be, as Doug Gourlay, MD, puts it, "talented amateurs" in addiction medicine. Educationally, physicians, nurses, psychologists and others frequently report that their training included little formal teaching about pain. Teaching about addiction lags behind even further. And training on the pain/addiction interface is almost non-existent. This volume goes headlong into the gaps in all of our education and training and goes a long way toward making up for the inadequacies mentioned above. I hope it becomes a staple of pain education and training and is used to teach the important practical aspects of proper opioid pain management to members of all disciplines, prescribers and non-prescribers, for years to come.

Steven D. Passik, PhD
Associate Attending Psychologist
Memorial Sloan Kettering Cancer Center
Associate Professor of Psychiatry
Weill College of Cornell Medical Center
New York, NY

ACKNOWLEDGMENTS

We would like to thank the study authors and pioneers in the fields of pain and addiction medicine whose work came before. We express appreciation to the editors at Sunrise River Press for their skill and support and to Ira Grunther for his fine work on illustrations. This book is dedicated to patients who battle twin demons of chronic pain and opioid abuse with a valor humbling to see.

INTRODUCTION

Compassion is not religious business, it is human business; it is not luxury,
it is essential ... for human survival.
- Tenzin Gyatso, the 14th Dalai Lama of Tibet[1]

Prescription drugs are newsworthy, particularly when they are abused in violation of their intended medical purpose. Conservative radio commentator Rush Limbaugh grabbed many headlines when he admitted his own misuse of the painkilling opium derivatives known as opioids. Limbaugh is only 1 of many famous abusers of prescription drugs, although he is perhaps the most surprising example, because his proposed solution to the widespread abuse problem before his own arrest was to convict drug abusers and "send them up the river."[2] The nonfamous are similarly afflicted, according to a study from Columbia University in New York, which found that prescription drugs (including opioids, stimulants, and depressants) had attracted 15.1 million admitted abusers by 2003.[3] That figure is double the number from only a decade earlier, and it includes more people than the total population of Tokyo. Today, only marijuana, alcohol, and tobacco are more popular than prescription agents as drugs of abuse. Of all prescriptions, opioids attract the most new abusers.[4]

However, opioids, which are so dangerous in the hands of abusers, are beneficial or even lifesaving for millions of people who otherwise would live with intractable pain. Nearly everyone seeks medical treatment to control pain at some point. Some will be unlucky enough to experience chronic pain that does not respond to treatment; about 70 million people live with chronic pain in America today.[5] In a world with few alternatives, opioids remain the best treatment available for many chronic pain conditions and are the first choice of therapy for acute and postoperative pain.

Clinicians who prescribe opioids to treat chronic pain are often caught between their professional obligation to relieve suffering and their desire to avoid contributing to the nonmedical consumption of controlled substances. Many medical practitioners fear becoming a source of medications that can be diverted for sale on the black market. They also dread the possibility of regulatory scrutiny or even prosecution that results from their patients' misuse of medication.

Thus the medical community is faced with a conundrum: Opioids offer safe, effective treatment for many chronic pain conditions and pose little risk of addiction for most patients who take them to control pain. However, some patients treated with opioids do display behaviors consistent with addiction. The challenge is to curtail the abuse and diversion of prescription opioids while ensuring their availability for patients who benefit from their use. The first step in resolving those seemingly conflicting interests is to acknowledge that they exist. Patients who suffer pain are often treated with prescribed painkilling drugs that can be abused. Because a certain segment of the opioid-treated pain population exhibits an active substance-use disorder, steps should be taken to minimize the very real potential for the abuse of such medications. The obligations to battle pain and addiction are not mutually exclusive, they are mutually inextricable.

This complex dilemma is summarized in the following list of the rights and responsibilities of healthcare professionals who prescribe opioids to treat pain (Box).[6] Although the task of safeguarding against substance abuse appears (and is) daunting, patients are not at equal risk for opioid addiction or abuse. The key to managing a patient's opioid intake lies in screening for abuse potential and carefully monitoring the progress of treatment. Those skills are within the capability of every caring, committed healthcare professional, even given the time constraints of practicing medicine in today's clinical settings.

Primary care physicians, nurse practitioners and other first-contact clinicians are uniquely positioned to make a difference at the beginning of medical treatment. Research indicates that a patient with chronic pain is far more likely to seek treatment from a family doctor or other healthcare professional than from a pain management specialist. Likewise, an individual struggling with a substance-use disorder is more often treated by a primary care physician than by a physician certified in addiction medicine. Those realities create an opportunity for first-contact clinicians to maximize the chances for success when patients begin opioid therapy.

"The bottom line is that there will never be enough specialists to deal with the problem," said Scott Fishman, MD, during his time as president of the American Academy of Pain Medicine, "so we have to train primary care physicians at the front lines to be able to do this as part of the basic care that we give patients."[7]

The medical obligations of physicians include:

• Treating pain adequately in all patients.
• Screening new patients for potential drug abuse or addiction.
• Monitoring patients' progress and addressing any harmful effects as they participate in opioid therapy.

Clinicians may receive little support in those endeavors. Medical schools provide scant training in either managing pain or treating addiction; most curricula are focused instead on teaching future doctors to recognize and eradicate disease. In a survey of physicians conducted by the Columbia University National Center on Addiction and Substance Abuse in New York, only 40% of the respondents had received any medical school training to help them identify prescription drug abuse or addiction in patients. Almost half of respondents said that they have difficulty discussing prescription drug abuse with their patients.[3] Pain management, which is a subject similarly neglected in many medical school curricula, consisted of only a few hours' instruction for the less than half of physicians who received any training. Even though some recent graduates of medical school indicate that training has improved in recent years, many physicians are still failing to diagnose active substance abuse, and medical students frequently graduate without having taken a single course on the treatment of pain. Furthermore, medical textbooks that address opioid abuse and chronic pain often refer to the topics separately. The complex interplay between substance abuse, mental disease, and chronic pain is rarely grasped or explored. In this book, we acknowledge the danger posed by the misuse of prescription opioids — a danger often downplayed by pain-control advocates. At the same time, we affirm the right of all people to be treated for pain. The latter perspective is sometimes ignored by addiction-treatment specialists.

We also assert with vigor that at no time should the guidelines presented here be taken as license to refuse to treat (or to undertreat) the pain of someone with a substance-use disorder. People who have problems managing drug intake experience acute, postsurgical, and chronic pain as often as do any other patients, and they are no less deserving of pain relief. The goal of providing good medical care is to improve the quality and duration of life for every patient. That goal is within reach; it simply requires a high level of professional concern and a strong commitment to monitoring patients' progress.

Policy and legal issues require attention from every prescriber of opioids. Because opioids can fall into the wrong hands, some policy makers want to solve the problem of substance abuse by banning certain agents from the U.S. market altogether. That solution is untenable, because some of the most frequently abused drugs are also the most effective against pain. Prohibition is not the answer to the problem of prescription drug abuse. Managing treatment with pharmaceutical analgesics is similar to managing an eating disorder. A person with problems managing food intake cannot solve the problem with abstinence, because eating is necessary for survival. Instead, that person's destructive impulses must be managed. Similarly, society cannot eliminate the use of opioids, even though they can harm

---

Rights and Responsibilities of Healthcare Professionals Who Prescribe Opioids to Treat Pain

- Pain is undertreated in part because healthcare professionals fear that patients may be harmed or that they themselves may incur regulatory, legal, or licensing penalties.
- The decision of whether to prescribe opioids is particularly difficult when a patient exhibits an addictive disorder or a risk factor for addiction.
- The decision to prescribe opioids must be made based on the healthcare professional's knowledge of the patient's medical and psychiatric conditions and response to treatment.
- The prescribing of opioids should not be deemed appropriate or inappropriate independent of such clinical knowledge.
- Healthcare professionals who prescribe opioids for pain may occasionally be misled by patients who wish to divert or misuse medications.
- Healthcare professionals who prescribe ongoing opioids have an obligation to understand the risks and management of addictive disease.
- Persistent failure to treat addiction is poor medical practice.
- Persistent failure to prescribe opioids effectively when their use is indicated is also poor medical practice.
- Physicians traditionally receive little or no education about pain management or the treatment of addiction.

Adapted from: American Academy of Pain Medicine, the American Pain Society, and the American Society of Addiction Medicine. Public policy statement on the rights and responsibilities of healthcare professionals in the use of opioids for the treatment of pain: A consensus document. Glenview, IL and Chevy Chase, MD; 2004.

some consumers. Like food, opioid analgesics are only as beneficial or as destructive as the motivations and compulsions of the user.

Opioids are not a cure-all, nor are they without significant risks for patients. However, opioids are used to control pain and improve function far more frequently than they serve as agents of destruction. The potential for prescription abuse is a challenge to be met and managed, not a reason to abandon pain management.

This book was written to help clinicians (including primary care physicians, nurse practitioners, psychiatrists, and others who treat pain) to sort out the clinical, regulatory, and ethical issues associated with the prescribing of opioid analgesics and to reduce the risk of medication misuse, abuse, and diversion. The recommendations presented here are based on the work of numerous experts in the fields of pain management and addiction. Although a book such as this can never be considered a complete treatise on those subjects, it can serve as a succinct and ready resource for clinicians. If knowledge is power, then the information published here is intended to instill the power and confidence needed for clinicians to safely treat their patients' pain and restore their dignity and lost quality of life. In that endeavor, knowledge is also compassion.

References

1. Tools for the study of Tibet: words for reflection. Global Source Education Web site. Available at: http://www.globalsourcenetwork.org/tibet_reflections.htm..Accessed April 8, 2007.
2. The Rush Limbaugh Show. Premiere Radio Networks. Oct. 5, 1995.
3. Under the Counter: The Diversion and Abuse of Controlled Prescription Drugs in the U.S. National Center on Addiction and Substance Abuse at Columbia University (CASA), New York, NY; 2005.
4. Substance Abuse and Mental Health Services Administration. (2006). Results from the 2005 National Survey on Drug Use and Health: National Findings (Office of Applied Studies, NSDUH Series H-30, DHHS Publication No. SMA 06-4194). Rockville, MD.
5. Rosenblum A, Joseph H, Fong C, Kipnis S, Cleland C, Portenoy RK. Prevalence and characteristics of chronic pain among chemically dependent patients in methadone maintenance and residential treatment facilities. JAMA. 2003 May 14;289(18):2370-8.
6. American Academy of Pain Medicine, the American Pain Society, and the American Society of Addiction Medicine. Public policy statement on the rights and responsibilities of healthcare professionals in the use of opioids for the treatment of pain: A consensus document. Glenview, IL and Chevy Chase, MD; 2004.
7. Wallis C. The right (and wrong) way to treat pain. Time Magazine. 2005; February 20.

CHAPTER I

OPIOID ABUSE:
PREVALENCE AND EPIDEMIOLOGY

I simply do not remember getting out of bed, being pulled over by the police,
or being cited for three driving infractions. That's not how I want to live my life,
and it's not how I want to represent the people of Rhode Island.
- Patrick Kennedy, US Congressman
On his way to the Mayo Clinic to seek help for addiction to prescription drugs.[1]

The abuse of prescription opioids is a real and increasing problem with steep costs to society and to individual patients. People abuse opioids for various reasons and not merely because they are addicted in a clinical sense. The failure to differentiate among common terms and definitions that pertain to substance-use disorders causes misunderstanding among physicians and patients. Clinicians should know that:

• Abuse and addiction are not synonymous.
• Abuse can usually be managed.
• Addiction can usually be predicted.

Fear of contributing to the abuse and illegal diversion for sale of these powerful medications is appropriate and should not be minimized. It is, however, possible to manage the risk while ensuring that opioids remain available for the many people who use them appropriately and benefit from them.

This chapter addresses the prevalence of opioid abuse in the United States and its relationship to chronic pain, and it provides an overview of the nomenclature common to the specialties of pain management and addiction. Armed with this knowledge, clinicians will be better positioned to recognize and address the various categories of problematic opioid use.

Prescription Abuse Is Increasing

Substance abuse is a leading cause of preventable illness and death in the United States.[2] The misuse of drugs ruins families, costs billions in lost productivity, strains the healthcare system, and ends lives.

Against this backdrop, prescription drugs are becoming the new substances of choice for many recreational drug users (Box I:1- Box I:2, Figure I:1). According to researchers at Columbia University, more Americans now abuse prescriptions than use cocaine, hallucinogens, inhalants, and heroin combined.[3] Opioid analgesics, tranquilizers, and stimulants are among the most frequently abused prescription drugs (Box I:3).

As the incidence of drug abuse skyrockets, more Americans every year are experimenting with the recreational use of prescription opioids for the first time. Many of those first-time users are young people.[4] Today, adolescents and people of college age appear caught in a cultural current in which prescription drug abuse is more accepted among peers than in the past (Box I:4). Older people are also at risk for substance abuse, particularly

Box 1:1

**Prescription Drug Abuse in America:
Columbia University Survey, 1992 – 2003**

• The number of Americans who admitted to abusing prescription drugs nearly doubled (from 7.8 million to 15.1 million).
• The number of people abusing prescription drugs increased 7 times faster than the increase in the US population.
• Prescription drug abuse among teenagers more than tripled.
• Almost 1 in 10 people who ranged in age from 12 to 17 years abused at least 1 controlled prescription drug in 2003.
• Controlled prescription drugs were implicated in 29.9% of drug-related emergency-room deaths (opioids accounted for 18.9% of those deaths) in 2002.

Source: Under the Counter: The Diversion and Abuse of Controlled Prescription Drugs in the U.S. National Center on Addiction and Substance Abuse at Columbia University (CASA), New York, NY; 2005.

death from overdose. Middle age is the most vulnerable time for death from accidental drug poisoning, according to data from medical examiners in several states.[5]

The increase in substance abuse has heightened social costs and the number of drug-related fatalities. Hospital emergency departments are feeling the strain from such incidents: Reports of overdose from narcotic analgesics rose 20% from 2001 to 2002, according to the U.S. Drug Abuse Warning Network.[6]

Box 1:2   **Current and New Nonmedical Users of Psychotherapeutic
Prescriptions in the United States, 2005**

An estimated 6.4 million people (2.6% of survey respondents age 12 years or older) used psychotherapeutic drugs nonmedically in the month before the survey.

• An estimated 4.7 million used pain relievers.
• 1.8 million used tranquilizers.
• 1.1 million used stimulants.
• 272,000 used sedatives.

"Nonmedical use of pain relievers" was the illicit drug category with the most new users (2.2 million) within the 12 months before the survey. The average age of new users was 21.2 years.

Source: Substance Abuse and Mental Health Services Administration. (2006). Results from the 2005 National Survey on Drug Use and Health: National Findings (Office of Applied Studies, NSDUH Series H-30, DHHS Publication No. SMA 06-4194). Rockville, MD.

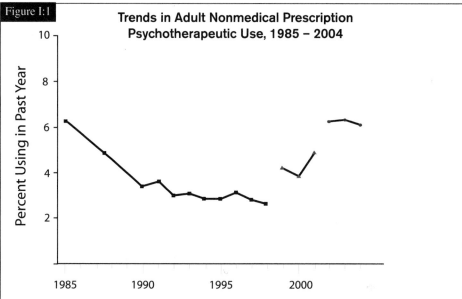

Figure I:1

Trends in Adult Nonmedical Prescription Psychotherapeutic Use, 1985 – 2004

Note: Data points represent surveys conducted since 1985. The 1985-1998 data are from NHSDA (PAPI), the 1999-2001 data are from NHSDA (CAI), and the 2002-2004 data are from NSDUH (CAI). The three series of NSDUH/NHSDA data use different methodologies and are not comparable with the other series.

Substance Abuse and Mental Health Services Administration. (2005). Results from the 2004 National Survey on Drug Use and Health: National Findings (Office of Applied Studies, NSDUH Series H-28, DHHS Publication No. SMA 05-4062). Rockville, MD.

The number of unintentional deaths from prescription drugs is also growing larger nationwide. In North Carolina between 1997 and 2001, deaths from illegal drugs decreased while deaths involving prescribed opioids increased 300%.[7] Other states are posting similar or even greater increases.[5] A federal study on drug-related mortality showed that opiates, including prescription pain relievers and heroin, were involved in deaths more often than any other type of drug in 29 of 32 metropolitan areas and in 6 states.[8]

Why Prescription Drugs, and Why Now?

Several reasons may contribute to the rising popularity of prescription drugs for recreational purposes. Such drugs are relatively easy to obtain. A convenient supply found in the family medicine cabinet has replaced the necessity for street procurement and its accompanying stigma. The Internet has ushered in the "age of the electronic pusher" in which Web sites advertise and sell controlled substances to anyone with a credit card, often without regard to the purchaser's prescription status or age.

Some experts believe that drugs of abuse are fads that are popular for a generation and then cycle out of fashion. Evidence shows that this may indeed be happening with respect to prescription drugs. The U.S. National Drug Intelligence Center reports that although prescription drug abuse climbed sharply during the 1990s, it appeared to have peaked by 2002[6] and has since leveled off.

Box 1:3	**Most-Abused Prescription Drugs**

• Opioids.

• Central nervous system depressants (used to treat anxiety and sleep disorders).

• Stimulants (used to treat attention-deficit hyperactivity disorder and narcolepsy).

Source: National Institute on Drug Abuse, National Institutes of Health, US Department of Health and Human Services. Abuse and Addiction, Research Report Series, *2005. NIH publication number 05-4881. Rockville, MD*

Certain drugs attain notoriety in the press, sometimes because of the involvement of law-enforcement agencies. Controlled-release oxycodone is one such opioid that has become a media sensation. When abusers circumvent the controlled-release formula of this or similar drugs by crushing tablets and then chewing, snorting, or injecting the powder, the result is the equivalent of 12 hours of medication delivered in a single "hit." Oxycodone abuse has spread in the United States and has generated publicity, particularly in rural areas and southern states.[9] Some attorneys have even begun trying to profit from media attention by running advertisements to recruit people treated with a prescribed drug who might want to seek restitution for the perceived fostering of addiction.

Any drug that is altered and consumed in defiance of medical direction has the potential to devastate lives. However, vilifying a brand-name drug that provides excellent analgesia for many compliant patients by applying nicknames such as "hillbilly heroin" confers to those treated the unfair stigma of implied drug abuse and encourages a certain societal complacency. If clinicians as a group conclude that prescription opioid abuse exists only in certain socioeconomic groups or in specific regions of the country, then they can remain uninvolved with issues of drug abuse. The resultant false sense of security obscures the truth: Any opioid can be abused in the hands of a determined and compulsive user.

A transdermal patch containing the potent opioid fentanyl is another narcotic pain reliever that has been associated with some deaths and is being closely watched by the U.S. Food and Drug Administration (FDA). The reasons for those deaths have not been established; however, fentanyl patches can be abused by extracting the medication intended for absorption through the skin and ingesting that form of the drug. Another delivery system of fentanyl also became a fad drug of abuse, although its popularity has not become a national problem. An analgesic lozenge that is absorbed through the oral mucous membranes to treat breakthrough pain and is dubbed the "perc-a-pop" by some recreational drug abusers appears to have special appeal to young people (Box I:5).

Regardless of the trends, no one (least of all ethical clinicians who treat pain) should underestimate the dangers posed by prescription drug abuse. However, it is important to distinguish between the illegal use of prescription opioids and the legal medical use of the same substances to treat pain. Media coverage and general public opinion often overlook a very important point: Most pain patients do not take analgesic medications to "get high." Every medication that can be abused is also a valuable tool for treating pain, often with few and manageable adverse effects.

Box 1:4	Prescription Drug Abuse in Young People

- About 1 in 5 teenagers has tried prescription painkillers to get high, according to the Partnership for a Drug-Free America.
- In 2004, more US teens had abused a prescription painkiller than Ecstasy, cocaine, crack, or lysergic acid diethylamide.

The most popular prescription drugs abused by US teens were:

- Hydrocodone (Vicodin) about 1 in 5 youths (18%).
- Oxycodone (OxyContin) (10%).
- Drugs for attention-deficit hyperactivity disorder, such as methylphenidate (Ritalin) or amphetamine and dextroamphetamine (Adderall) (10%).
- Only 48% of teens said they saw "great risk" in experimenting with prescription medicines.
- "Ease of access" was cited as a major factor in trying prescription medications for recreational purposes.
- A medicine cabinet at home or at a friend's home was a likely source of prescription medications for recreational use.

"A new category of substance abuse is emerging in America. Increasingly, teenagers are getting high through the intentional abuse of medications. In other words, Generation Rx has arrived."

Roy J. Bostock, Chairman of The Partnership for a Drug-Free America

Source: Generation Rx: National Study Reveals New Category of Substance Abuse Emerging: Teens Abusing Rx and OTC Medications Intentionally to Get High. Partnership for a Drug-Free America Web site. http://www.drugfree.org/Portal/About/NewsReleases/Teens_Abusing_Rx_and_OTC_Medications. Accessed April 8, 2007.

Chronic Pain

Some pain does not resolve after the original injury or site of surgery has healed. Pain accounts for 80% of all doctor visits,[10] and the most unfortunate patients experience chronic intractable pain. Left unchecked, chronic nonmalignant pain can erode independence and mobility, damage career and family relationships, and cost at least $61.2 billion a year in lost productivity.[11] The cost in diminished quality of life is incalculable.

When is pain defined as chronic? Definitions vary, but in general, pain is considered chronic if it is persistent (it can be intermittent) and if the cause cannot be removed.

Chronic pain:
- Persists longer than 3 or 6 months (opinions vary) and may continue unabated for weeks, months, or years.
- Persists beyond the normal healing process.
- Occurs after injury or may have no apparent cause.
- May spread beyond the original site of injury.

• Appears to serve no biological purpose.
• Is of moderate-to-severe intensity.
• Limits physiologic function.
• Impacts psychologic and emotional function.
• Significantly interferes with daily activities.
• Reduces quality of life.
• Is refractory to treatment.

Box 1:5

Perc-a-Pop

Used to refer to fentanyl in lozenge form.
Nickname originated in Philadelphia, Pennsylvania.
Most buyers are teenagers in Philadelphia.
Sold on streets for about $20 per dose.
Easy to abuse, sweet, has high appeal for young people.
Abuse appears isolated; national abuse rates are growing but remain relatively low:
• 576 incidents of nonmedical use in 2000
• 1506 incidents of nonmedical use in 2002

Source: Scolforo M. Abuse of narcotic "perc-a-pops" reported in Philadelphia. Associated Press. April 28, 2004.

Prevalence of Chronic Pain in America

After considering the results of an international survey of almost 26,000 primary care patients, Rosenblum and colleagues suggested in 2003 that 70 million U.S. adults live with chronic pain.[12] According to a survey conducted for the American Pain Society, approximately 9% of the U.S. adult population experiences moderate-to- severe pain.[13] Chronic nonmalignant pain is difficult to treat because it is often refractory to conventional treatment. Long-term therapy with opioids can bring a degree of relief and a return of function to many chronic-pain patients.

Opioids are synthetic compounds that are similar in structure and action to the natural opiates derived from the poppy plant (Box I:6). Opioids bind to receptors in the brain and spinal cord as do endorphins (the body's natural analgesics). Thus opioids inhibit pain transmission by blocking the sensation of pain that is conveyed by nerve cells. Opioid treatment rarely produces complete relief from pain. However, a review of the literature revealed that patients with chronic nonmalignant pain experienced a significant improvement in function and quality of life as a result of long-term opioid therapy.[14] Chronic pain may even be

Box 1:6

Opioids Often Prescribed to Treat Pain

• Codeine.
• Fentanyl.
• Hydrocodone.
• Hydromorphone.
• Levorphanol.
• Meperidine.
• Methadone.
• Morphine.
• Morphine sustained-release.
• Oxycodone.
• Oxycodone controlled-release.

preventable if it is treated aggressively and early. For that reason, it is vital that common fears and misconceptions associated with the prescribing of opioids not be allowed to cloud treatment choices.

Chronic Pain Meets Fear of Opioids

The treatment of chronic nonmalignant pain presents a far more difficult clinical challenge than does therapy for acute or postoperative pain. The use of opioids is most controversial in patients with chronic nonmalignant pain, mainly because clinicians often fear that prescribing opioids could contribute to drug abuse or addiction. The fear that patients are faking some or all of their pain symptoms just to obtain narcotic pain medication causes some clinicians to stigmatize the use of opioids and to mislabel pain patients as addicts. This presents, perhaps, the greatest single barrier to the availability of pain relief. To a somewhat lesser degree, clinicians also fear regulatory or legal action connected with the prescribing of opioids and the induction of obtundation or oversedation in patients who are treated with opioids.

Cognitive tests performed in patients treated with opioids have shown that the agents produce little to no reduction in cognitive function.[15] Any sedation or impairment that does occur tends to develop in patients whose opioid therapy has just begun. Over time, those adverse effects of opioid treatment nearly always resolve.

Clinicians' common concern about "creating drug addicts" or otherwise increasing the societal problem with prescription drug abuse is understandable, but when such fears are allowed to drive decisions concerning pain management, patients suffer. Consider the following case:

> A patient was suffering severe pain because of complications after plastic surgery. The surgeon who performed her surgery refused to treat her pain with opioid analgesics because he feared losing his medical license. The patient was subsequently referred to a pain specialist who prescribed strong opioids that were required for only 2 weeks.

When physicians agree to perform surgery but then refuse to treat postoperative pain, their fear of prescribing opioids has become exaggerated. The refusal to adequately relieve postsurgical pain is unconscionable. Protection against legal penalties after prescribing opioids will be covered in greater detail in a later chapter. It should be noted, however, that opioids are controlled substances, and the government tracks their use closely. Careful documentation and familiarization with federal and state laws pertaining to opioids are the best tools clinicians can use to protect themselves and their practices.

Regardless of how experienced or careful the clinician, he or she will likely be fooled at some time by a patient seeking opioids for sale or for a nonmedical purpose. However, those individuals represent a minority, and far too many patients who require opioids to relieve severe pain are stigmatized as "drug seekers." Most patients seek relief from their pain and nothing more. Ways to avoid becoming the instrument of diverters will be outlined later in this book.

The Importance of Treating Pain

Out-of-control pain does not make the patient stronger from the suffering it induces; it destroys health and well-being. Researchers have found that malignant tumor growth is slowed by the administration of painkillers.[16] Pain inhibits the body's immune system and impacts heart rate, blood pressure, and respiration. Pain that persists and becomes chronic rewires the body's nervous system to continue sending signals even after the original cause has healed or been removed. Subsequent damage to neural pathways can be permanent. Anxiety, depression, and insomnia make the pain doubly unbearable.

Fortunately, the last decade has brought greater emphasis on pain management and frequent calls for supportive pain-control guidelines and public policies. A spotlight focused on the issues in the summer of 2000, when the US Congress passed a bill designating a "Decade of Pain Control and Research." In January 2001, US hospitals were required to implement new standards from the Joint Commission on Accreditation of Healthcare Organizations to improve pain assessment and management. One of the standards requires healthcare professionals to consider pain as an entity separate from its cause. Pain became designated the "fifth vital sign" in addition to the other vital signs (body temperature, pulse, respiration, and blood pressure). Although these encouraging signs suggest that the serious detriment of pain is being recognized, the number of people who are undertreated for pain still far outstrips the segment of the population afflicted by drug abuse.[17]

In these pages, our focus is to acknowledge and address the drug-related behaviors that sometimes compromise pain treatment with opioids. For that reason, little space has been devoted to the appropriate clinical methods of pain management, such as initiating and changing doses or providing alternative pain therapies if opioid treatment becomes inadvisable for a given patient. Several good pain-management guides are available. A couple of recommendations for clinicians are *A Clinical Guide to Opioid Analgesia* by authors Fine and Portenoy, published by McGraw-Hill,[18] and *The Pain EDU.org Manual: A Clinical Companion* by Menefee and Katz published by Inflexxion, Inc.[19] Both are available online.

A History of Opium and Opioid Use

The history of opiates as instruments of pain relief has spanned millennia and produced many consequences, some good and some less than desirable. The use of opium harkens back at least to ancient Sumeria (c 3400 BC) and was known among the Egyptians in 1300 BC.[20] Although Hippocrates (c 460 BC) recognized the usefulness of opium as a painkilling narcotic, it was often consumed to produce euphoria for purely recreational purposes. The psychogenic effects proved very popular among 19th century writers such as John Keats and Elizabeth Barrett Browning.

The 19th century also brought 2 developments of immense medical significance: the isolation of morphine (the active ingredient in opium), which was termed "God's own medicine," and the invention of the hypodermic needle. However, as the 20th century dawned, opiates began to fall out of favor as addiction fears grew and the US government assumed legal control of the prescribing and dispensing of controlled substances.

The distrust of narcotics sometimes extended even to the practice of refusing sufficient medication to ease pain. The belief grew that pain, particularly if it is endured without complaint, fosters character. In the 1940s, the *British Medical Journal* quoted a respected practitioner who downplayed the importance of newly available anesthetics to ease childbirth pain.[21] He reasoned that mothers whose childbirth was not painful might cease to love their children.

In the United States, much needless suffering resulted from the "stiff upper lip" approach to medical care. Yet as the progress of scientific inquiry took hold, that attitude began to change. With the discovery of opiate receptors in the central nervous system, acceptance slowly was reignited for the administration of opioids sufficient to treat acute and postsurgical pain and the ongoing pain caused by cancer. Even so, the use of opioids to ease chronic nonmalignant pain continued to be frowned upon by the medical establishment and was sometimes even prosecuted by law.

A new era of greater pain control dawned in the late 1980s and gained in popularity throughout the 1990s. It was then that the widespread acceptance of opioids used to treat chronic nonmalignant pain grew in part as a result of numerous studies that reported the undertreatment of pain to be common and analgesia-induced addiction rare. As a hallmark of the increasing acceptance of analgesics used to control pain, a 1997 consensus document published by the American Academy of Pain Medicine and the American Pain Society advised all types of clinicians (not just specialists) to consider the use of opioids in selected patients for the management of chronic nonmalignant pain.[22] During that time, pain-control advocates, who were eager to heal the scourge of undertreated pain, may have underestimated the risk of abuse posed by opioid therapy. In recent years, those same advocates have begun to sound a cautionary note. One such expert is Russell K. Portenoy, MD, a pioneer and preeminent leader in pain management. In an Australian radio interview about the fight against chronic pain, Portenoy said he was embarrassed by his own minimization of the risk of drug abuse when he taught other clinicians how to use opioids to treat chronic pain 10 years earlier.[23] He said, "I did that because I thought that in patients with chronic pain, these risks could be minimized, and that compared with the problem of undertreated pain, the concern about abuse, addiction, and diversion was not that relevant. Fast-forward 10 years later, and we recognize that was a big error."[23]

This brief overview of the use of analgesic agents brings us to the present day, when the extent of the solution must parallel the size of the problem. As Portenoy said, "Doctors have to have two sets of skills to use these drugs safely and effectively, or they shouldn't use them." Those sets of skills are prescribing opioids and minimizing the risk of abuse.

Prevalence of Addiction in Chronic-Pain Patients

The prevalence of addiction in pain patients has almost certainly been underestimated in the recent past. In truth, the prevalence of drug abuse and addiction in patients treated with opioids for chronic pain has not been established because of the lack of prospective studies. Most research indicates that patients with chronic pain tend to abuse substances, including alcohol, at estimated rates of 10% to 18%, which are similar to or slightly higher than those in the general U.S. population.[24-25] About 1% of the general U.S. population demonstrates addiction to opioids.[26] At least 1 study has shown that 2% to 5% of chronic-pain patients manifest addiction (a rate more than twice that of the general population).[27]

However, the extent to which opioids prescribed for pain actively foster an addiction that did not already exist has sometimes been exaggerated, particularly in the popular imagination. According to the results of a survey of 1000 American adults in 2002, most (78%) believed that treating pain with strong medicines is very likely or somewhat likely to result in addiction.[28] Only 1 in 5 respondents thought the likelihood of addiction to be low. Although abuse, addiction, and diversion are serious issues in a minority of patients who exhibit those problems, research clearly indicates that most patients treated with prescribed opioids for acute or chronic pain will not become addicted to their medication.

Patients with a history of substance abuse and poor social support who are not in a recovery program and who are receiving long-term opioid therapy are at high risk for abusing their medication, whether or not that abuse reflects true addiction.[29] However, even patients with a history of substance abuse are not destined to abuse prescribed opioids if they are adequately monitored and receive sufficient support. Whatever the true addiction rate in US chronic-pain patients, it is the risk of addiction or abuse in each individual patient that is of greatest concern to clinicians. Guidelines for assessing the potential for opioid abuse in individual patients are outlined in a later chapter.

When Pain Is the Problem

Chronic-pain patients who receive long-term opioid therapy often face deep resistance to their treatment from family members, friends, and employers who view those patients with suspicion. One such patient was in stable condition and her pain was well controlled by opioid medication for more than 20 years. Nevertheless, she was pleased when a newer pain-control method – a spinal implant that delivers medication – allowed her to reduce the number of tablets she took. When she shared this information, her sister took the opportunity to vent a long-held belief: "I always knew you were an addict." A lack of understanding about addiction leads to demeaning statements like this one. Incidents such as these are humiliating for pain patients and occur far too frequently.

Box 1:7   **Characteristics of Chronic-Pain Patients Versus Addicted Patients**

Chronic-Pain Patient

- Medication use is not out of control.
- Medication use improves quality of life.
- Wants to decrease medication if adverse effects develop.
- Is concerned about the physical problem that is being treated with the drug.
- Follows the agreement for the use of the opioid.
- Frequently has leftover medication.

Addicted Patient

- Medication use is out of control.
- Medication use causes a diminished quality of life.
- Medication use continues or increases despite adverse effects.
- Unaware of or in denial about any problems that develop as a result of drug treatment.
- Does not follow the agreement for the use of the opioid.
- Does not have leftover medication, loses prescriptions, always has a "story" about why additional drug treatment is necessary.

Much confusion abounds regarding what causes addiction (Box I:7). Some clinicians believe they have turned a patient into an addict if that patient displays symptoms of tolerance to an opioid medication. Far too many people believe that a family member is addicted because he or she "looks drunk." Because the nomenclature available to today's practicing clinicians does not always adequately reflect the reality observed in the patients they treat, the lexicon used most commonly to refer to opioid use should be reviewed.

Definitions Associated with Opioid Use and Abuse

Inadequate or misused terminology can limit the ability to speak with clarity and ac-

---

Box 1:8

Definitions Associated with Opioid Use and Abuse

Abuse

The use of any substance for a nontherapeutic purpose or the use of medication for purposes other than those for which the agent is prescribed.

Addiction

A primary chronic neurobiologic disease influenced by genetic, psychosocial, and environmental factors. It is characterized by impaired control over drug use, compulsive drug use, and continued drug use despite harm and because of craving.

Tolerance

A physiologic state caused by the regular use of an opioid in which increased doses are needed to maintain the same effect. In patients with "analgesic tolerance," increased doses of the opioid are needed to maintain pain relief.

Physical Dependence

A physiologic state characterized by abstinence syndrome (withdrawal) if treatment with an opioid is stopped or decreased abruptly or an opioid antagonist is administered. It is an expected result of opioid therapy and does not by itself equal addiction.

Abstinence Syndrome (Withdrawal)

A syndrome characterized by symptoms that include sweating, tremor, vomiting, anxiety, insomnia, and muscle pain. Abstinence syndrome is caused by a reduction in the opioid dose or the administration of an opioid antagonist. It can be avoided by carefully tapering the opioid dosage and monitoring the patient.

Definitions adapted from the following sources:

American Academy of Pain Medicine, American Pain Society, and American Society of Addiction Medicine. Definitions related to the use of opioids for the treatment of pain: consensus document. Under review. Glenview, IL and Chevy Chase, MD; 2001.

Federation of State Medical Boards of the United States. Model policy for the use of controlled substances for the treatment of pain. Available at: http://www.fsmb.org/pdf/2004_grpol_Controlled_Substances.pdf. Accessed April 10, 2007.

curacy about substance-use disorders. To counteract such confusion, clinicians should give thorough consideration to what is meant by terms like "addiction," "abuse," "tolerance," and "physical dependence" (Box I:8). Such terms are frequently misunderstood in clinical circles, in casual conversations, in media accounts, by well-meaning friends and family members of patients, and by patients themselves.

The differences in meaning of terms that pertain to opioid use are important. A person who is physically dependent on a drug, for example, may experience symptoms of withdrawal if treatment with that drug is suddenly interrupted or terminated. Such symptoms do not in themselves indicate addiction. Similarly, a person who aggressively demands more medication may be suffering from undertreated pain and not from addiction. The following definitions are derived from several sources (primarily the 2001 consensus document titled *Definitions Related to the Use of Opioids for the Treatment of Pain*, which has been endorsed by the American Academy of Pain Medicine, the American Pain Society, and the American Society of Addiction Medicine).[30]

Physical Dependence

This is one of the most frequently misunderstood and misapplied terms. "Physical dependence" is often misinterpreted as referring to addiction. Instead, it is a natural physiologic response to the persistent use of opioids. Physical dependence merely means that the body has adapted to the blood level of the opioid in the system and that the patient is likely to exhibit symptoms of abstinence syndrome, otherwise known as "withdrawal," if treatment with the drug is abruptly terminated or sharply decreased or if an opioid antagonist is administered.

Some of the confusion over the term "dependence" stems from definitions contained in the *Diagnostic and Statistical Manual of Mental Disorders, Fourth Edition, Text Revised (DSM-IV-TR)*.[31] The *DSM-IV-TR* defines substance dependence, including opioid dependence, as essentially synonymous with addiction; it fails to distinguish between the disease of chemical dependence and the natural physiologic response of physical dependence. The *DSM-IV-TR* even goes so far as to list tolerance and withdrawal symptoms among the "defining features" of addiction (substance dependence), thus further impeding the chances of differentiating a true disease process from a normal physiologic reaction.

It is essential to use correct terms to refer to medical and nonmedical opioid consumption. A person who is addicted to an opioid medication may also be physically dependent on that agent. However, an addicted person will not only exhibit abstinence syndrome if treatment with the opioid is stopped but will also display a lack of control over the use of the drug, compulsive use of the agent, craving for the drug, and continued use despite harm, all of which are hallmarks of addiction. Furthermore, the absence of physical dependence does not mean that a person is not addicted. Cocaine is an example of a strongly addicting substance that does not, when the drug is suddenly stopped, cause the type of withdrawal that opioids do. Thus cocaine is not a strong catalyst for physical dependence, but thousands of ruined lives attest to its addictive power.

Physical dependence can occur with drugs other than opioids. Treatment with certain anticonvulsants and antidepressants, for example, also cannot be stopped abruptly without inducing abstinence syndrome, yet those medications are not associated with addiction. Although abstinence syndrome does not develop when treatment with insulin is quickly withdrawn, insulin is necessary for physical function and a good quality of life in some diabetic individuals. In that regard, some diabetic patients can be said to be dependent on insulin. In a similar manner, analgesics increase physical function and improve the quality of life for patients with chronic pain, even if opioid therapy is maintained long term and the opioid doses seem massive to laypeople.

When opioids become unnecessary because pain has resolved, dosages should be carefully and slowly tapered to avoid abstinence syndrome. Guidelines for discontinuing opioid therapy are provided in Chapter VI. The patient should be monitored closely for the development of clinical symptoms. Some patients are very sensitive to the withdrawal process and will require pharmacologic treatment. This tapering of medication is not equal to "detoxing" the patient, because the patient is not toxic if he or she is taking medication only to avoid withdrawal. Experts in pain management and the treatment of addiction prefer the term "transitioning."

To recap, physical dependence is:
- A normal physiologic state.
- An expected result of opioid use.
- Characterized by withdrawal (abstinence syndrome) if treatment with the opioid is suddenly terminated or decreased or if an opioid antagonist is given.
- Highly variable in its onset, depending on the individual patient.
- A phenomenon that sometimes coincides with addiction.
- Is not, by itself, an indication of addiction.

Tolerance

Like physical dependence, tolerance is a natural physiologic response to regular opioid use. Tolerance is defined as the need to increase an opioid dose to maintain the same effect or, if the dose is kept constant, a reduction in effect. The effects of opioids include those that are wanted, such as analgesia, and those that are unwanted, such as respiratory depression, sedation, nausea, constipation, and a reinforcing action on the brain's "reward center," which poses the danger of addiction. The rate at which tolerance to the various effects of opioids develops varies among patients.

Analgesic tolerance, or the need to increase the opioid dose to achieve the same level of pain relief, is not a sign of addiction, nor is it considered a factor that contributes to the risk of addiction. Not every individual experiences analgesic tolerance. Great variations exist in the individual response to opioids, just as pain perception varies greatly among individuals. Research shows that younger people develop tolerance more quickly (and thus need more frequent dose adjustments) than do older individuals.[32]

There is no arbitrary ceiling beyond which a dose of opioids is unsafe. Clinicians who treat chronic pain are able to administer large doses of opioids to opioid-tolerant patients; the same doses would be unsafe in opioid-naïve patients. Therefore, a physician cannot be said to be "overprescribing" opioids solely on the basis of the quantity and frequency of prescribing. Sometimes, more opioids are needed to treat pain because the patient's disease has worsened. Some patients may need more medication to treat pain caused by increased activity because their physical functioning has improved. Those types of dose titrations are not associated with tolerance.

In summary, tolerance:
• Is a natural state of neuroadaptation to drug-induced changes.
• May result in increased analgesic needs.
• Develops at different rates for different effects such as analgesia, sedation and nausea.
• Varies among individuals.
• Varies according to the type of pain.
• Develops more quickly in younger people than in older individuals.
• Is not addiction.

Tolerance begins to develop immediately after the first ingestion of an opioid. Only a few days of opioid therapy can lead to some degree of tolerance and physical dependence. Patients who receive short-term opioid treatment can experience mild flu-like symptoms when therapy with the drug is stopped. For most patients treated with opioids, these are manageable adverse effects of therapy. Patients with chronic nonmalignant pain who experience good analgesia with opioid therapy should not be deprived of pain relief because of those effects.

Abuse

The definitions or criteria for substance abuse include:
• Intentional overuse of the substance during periods of celebration, anxiety, or despair or as a result of self-medication or ignorance.
• A maladaptive pattern of substance use that leads to clinically significant impairment or distress.
• The use of any substance for a nontherapeutic purpose.
• The use of a medication outside the scope of usual medical practice.
• When the abuse of prescribed opioids is described, the best definition is probably that provided by the US Substance Abuse and Mental Health Services Administration: "any nonmedical use of a substance."

If abuse is defined as any use of a medication in defiance of medical direction, then abuse is a very widespread phenomenon indeed, and it encompasses a nearly infinite variety of behaviors and motivations. A few of the reasons why abuse occurs include:

• Experimentation.
• To escape stress or boredom.
• Peer norms.
• To manage anxiety or depression.
• To mitigate a comorbid mental disorder.
• To mask unhappiness stemming from life's problems, whether marital, financial, health, or other.
• To curb undertreated pain.
• Addiction.

The lifelong heroin addict is an abuser. So is the person who, when trying to conserve finances, consumes his wife's prescription opioids on only 1 occasion because he has a toothache.

Drug abuse is often confused with addiction, which is a medical condition that also involves the misuse of substances. There is a crucial distinction, however: Abuse that does not stem from addiction tends to decrease when adverse consequences (legal, social, or physical) begin to worsen the individual's life.

It is important to understand that:
• Abusers may or may not also be addicted.
• Abusers can often stop when harm occurs.

What exactly are the adverse consequences of medication abuse? The 2001 consensus statement[30] on opioid prescribing details some of them:
• Persistent sedation or intoxication resulting from overuse.
• Increasing functional impairment.
• Medical complications.
• Psychologic manifestations such as irritability, apathy, anxiety, or depression.
• Legal problems.
• Economic problems.
• Social problems.

Patients who misuse their medications may experience some of the above characteristics and still may not be addicted. Many possible reasons can drive prescription drug abuse, some of which will be explored later. Some cases of ongoing, egregious, or intractable abuse do indeed require the release of a patient from care — a process that must be accomplished according to legal and ethical guidelines. However, abuse is a common occurrence and can usually be managed by clinical interventions.

Addiction

Tolerance and physical dependence are expected physiologic effects of opioid therapy; addiction is not. Addiction is a chronic primary disease with a neurobiologic basis. Unlike abusers who can stop the abuse when harm occurs, addicted people so crave the substance they abuse that they are willing to sacrifice every aspect of their lives rather than do without that substance. Health, marriage, career, reputation, and financial status can crumble into ruin, but the addicted person cannot stop seeking the substance that is causing the destruction. A person with addictive disease is likely also to be physically dependent on the drug, and he or she is at high risk for the recurrence of addiction even after detoxification has been accomplished.

Addiction is characterized by the following behaviors, which are known as the "4C's:"
• Impaired control over drug use
• Compulsive use of the drug
• Continued use of the drug despite harm (physical, mental, and/or social)
• Craving for the drug

People with addictive disease may feel euphoric or "high" after taking an opioid. It is that euphoric experience or some other psychogenic reward that leads them to seek and re-seek the substance to which they are addicted. It should be noted that patients without the disease of addiction are more likely than addicted patients to experience an unpleasant re-action to an opioid prescribed for pain. That said, the experience of a pleasurable feeling is sometimes simply an effect of taking opioid medications and does not, in itself, indicate that an individual has become addicted.

Drug-produced euphoria does not produce the disease of addiction. Most people ex-posed to a substance with addictive properties do not become addicted to that substance. Co-caine, for example, which is one of the world's most addictive drugs, induces true chemical dependence in only 16% of its users.[33] Opioid medications may trigger or retrigger addic-tion in individuals who exhibit a complex interplay of vulnerabilities, but medications do not cause addiction. If this were true, every patient who received a medication with addic-tive potential would become addicted to that drug.

It should also be noted that a patient with a history of addictive disease or a vulnera-bility that indicates the potential for addictive disease experiences pain, both chronic and acute, as frequently as does any other patient. Patients who are vulnerable to addiction de-serve pain treatment, too, and they are at particular risk for having their pain ignored or minimized.

Abuse behaviors can indicate the presence of the disease of addiction, or they can in-dicate another underlying problem, such as undertreated pain or the presence of a mental dis-order. More discussion on the many different possible triggers of medication abuse, some of which closely mimic addiction, will follow in Chapter III.

Conclusion

Prescription opioid abuse is a growing phenomenon that no ethical health practitioner can ignore. The correct use of language will help clinicians and patients to more precisely identify and address the various clinical conditions related to pain and the use of opioids. "Abuse" is not necessarily "addiction," nor should "addiction" be confused with other terms such as "tolerance" or "physical dependence," both of which are expected physiologic re-sponses to opioid consumption.

References

1. Text of Patrick Kennedy's statement. The Associated Press. May 5, 2006.
2. Stewart WF, Ricci JA, Chee E, Morganstein D, Lipton R. Lost productive time and cost due to common pain conditions in the US workforce. JAMA. 2003 Nov 12;290(18):2443-54.
3. Under the Counter: The Diversion and Abuse of Controlled Prescription Drugs in the U.S. National Center on Addiction and Substance Abuse at Columbia University (CASA), New York, NY; 2005.
4. Generation Rx: National Study Reveals New Category of Substance Abuse Emerging: Teens Abusing Rx and OTC Medications Intentionally to Get High. Partnership for a Drug-Free   America   Web   site.   Available   at:

http://www.drugfree.org/Portal/About/NewsReleases/Teens_Abusing_Rx_and_OTC_
Medications. Accessed April 8, 2007.

5. Centers for Disease Control and Prevention (CDC). Unintentional and undetermined poisoning deaths—11 states, 1990-2001. MMWR Morb Mortal Wkly Rep. 2004 Mar 26;53(11):233-8.

6. National Drug Intelligence Center. Pharmaceuticals: Drug Threat Assessment. US Department of Justice. Product No. 2004-L0487-001. November 2004.

7. North Carolina Department of Health and Human Services. Findings and recommendations of the task force to prevent deaths from unintentional drug overdoses in North Carolina, 2003. (Division of Public Health, Injury and Violence Prevention Branch). Raleigh, NC.

8. Substance Abuse and Mental Health Services Administration, Office of Applied Studies. Drug Abuse Warning Network, 2003: Area Profiles of Drug-Related Mortality. DAWN Series D-27, DHHS Publication No. (SMA) 05-4023. Rockville, MD, 2005.

9. Hays LR. A profile of OxyContin addiction. J Addict Dis 2004; 23(4):1-9.

10. The Arthritis Foundation Pain In America: Highlights from a Gallup Survey, 2000. Arthritis   Foundation   Web   site.   Available   at: http://www.arthritis.org/conditions/speakingofpain/factsheet.asp. Accessed March 1, 2004.

11. Stewart WF, Ricci JA, Chee E, Morganstein D, Lipton R. Lost productive time and cost due to common pain conditions in the US workforce. JAMA. 2003 Nov 12;290(18):2443-54.

12. Rosenblum A, Joseph H, Fong C, Kipnis S, Cleland C, Portenoy RK. Prevalence and characteristics of chronic pain among chemically dependent patients in methadone maintenance and residential treatment facilities. JAMA. 2003 May 14;289(18):2370-8.

13. Roper Starch Worldwide, Inc. Chronic Pain In America: Roadblocks To Relief. Research conducted for the American Pain Society, the American Academy of Pain Medicine and Janssen Pharmaceutica, Jan. 1999. American Pain Society Web site. Available at: http://www.ampainsoc.org/whatsnew/conclude_road.htm. Accessed March 2, 2004.

14. Devulder J, Richarz U, Nataraja SH. Impact of long-term use of opioids on quality of life in patients with chronic, non-malignant pain. Curr Med Res Opin. 2005 Oct;21(10):1555-68.

15. Ersek M, Cherrier MM, Overman SS, Irving GA. The cognitive effects of opioids. Pain Manag Nurs. 2004;Jun;5(2):75-93.

16. Jiang Y, Weinberg J, Wilkinson DA, Emerman JT. Effects of steroid hormones and opioid peptides on the growth of androgen-responsive Shionogi carcinoma (SC115) cells in primary culture. Cancer Res 1993 Sep 15;53(18):4224-9.

17. Douglas E. Clinicians underestimate pain, resulting in undertreatment. Anesthesiology News. 2005 April;31(4).

18. Fine PG, Portenoy RK. A Clinical Guide to Opioid Analgesia. Minneapolis, MN: McGraw-Hill; 2004.

19. Menefee L, Katz N. The Pain EDU.org Manual: A Clinical Companion. Newton, MA: Inflexxion, Inc., 2003.

20. Booth M. Opium: A History. 1st US ed.. New York, NY: Thomas Dunne Books; 1998.
21. Without pain. Time Magazine. 1948; June 28.
22. American Academy of Pain Medicine and American Pain Society. The use of opioids for the treatment of chronic pain: A consensus statement. Glenview, IL; 1997.
23. A world of pain. ABC Radio National – Background Briefing. Produced by Helen Thomas. Dec. 5, 2004.
24. Savage SR. Assessment for addiction in pain-treatment settings. Clin J Pain. 2002 Jul-Aug;18(4 Suppl):S28-38.
25. Weaver M, Schnoll S. Abuse liability in opioid therapy for pain treatment in patients with an addiction history. Clin J Pain. 2002 Jul-Aug;18(4 Suppl):S61-9.
26. Robinson RC, Gatchel RJ, Polatin P, Deschner M, Noe C, Gajraj N. Screening for problematic prescription opioid use. Clin J Pain. 2001 Sep;17(3):220-8.
27. Webster LR, Webster RM. Predicting aberrant behaviors in opioid-treated patients: preliminary validation of the Opioid Risk Tool. Pain Med. 2005 Nov-Dec;6(6):432-42.
28. American Chronic Pain Association. Pain Awareness Is Important to Nurses. Pain Awareness Survey, June 2002. Partners for Understanding Pain [tool kit], September 2003. Rocklin, CA: American Chronic Pain Association; 2003.
29. Dunbar SA, Katz NP. Chronic opioid therapy for nonmalignant pain in patients with a history of substance abuse: report of 20 cases. J Pain Symptom Manage. 1996 Mar;11(3):163-71.
30. American Academy of Pain Medicine, American Pain Society, and American Society of Addiction Medicine. Definitions related to the use of opioids for the treatment of pain: consensus document. Under review. Glenview, IL and Chevy Chase, MD; 2001.
31. American Psychiatric Association, ed. Diagnostic and Statistical Manual of Mental Disorders. 4th ed, text revised (DSM-IV). Washington, DC: American Psychiatric Association; 2000.
32. Buntin-Mushock C, Phillip L, Moriyama K, Palmer PP. Age-dependent opioid escalation in chronic pain patients. Anesth Analg. 2005 Jun;100(6):1740-5.
30. American Academy of Pain Medicine, American Pain Society, and American Society of Addiction Medicine. Definitions related to the use of opioids for the treatment of pain: consensus document. Under review. Glenview, IL and Chevy Chase, MD; 2001.
33. O'Brien CP, Gardner EL. Critical assessment of how to study addiction and its treatment: human and non-human animal models. Pharmacol Ther. 2005 Oct;108(1):18-58.

CHAPTER II

THE NEUROBIOLOGY OF ADDICTION

There are more television addicts, more baseball and football addicts,
more movie addicts, and certainly more alcohol addicts in this country than
there are narcotics addicts.
- Shirley Chisholm, former US congresswoman
Testimony to House Select Committee on Crime, September 17, 1969[1]

People who abuse opioids are not necessarily addicted, but because addiction is a progressive disease that can be fatal if not arrested, it deserves a special focus. Until recently, addiction has been viewed as a volitional behavior stemming from weakness of character. Society frequently criminalizes the behaviors associated with addiction and does not treat those behaviors as manifestations of a medical disease. Our legal system reflects this pervasive attitude by incarcerating drug abusers without adequate substance-abuse treatment, although extensive data demonstrate the neurobiologic basis of addiction and indicate that the disease requires a medical solution.

For that reason, it is important to consider the overview of the neurobiology of addiction. That subject could be approached from a variety of perspectives. We have chosen to divide the discussion into 3 main areas: the major neuroanatomic structures that contribute to addiction, the communication pathways between those sites that facilitate the disease, and the neurochemical molecular changes that occur in the brain of long-term opioid abusers.

Box	Risk of Addiction by Type of Substance*		
	Ever used (%)	Dependence (%)	Risk (%)
Tobacco	75.6	24.1	31.9
Cocaine	16.2	2.7	16.7
Heroin	1.5	0.4	23.1
Stimulant	15.3	1.7	11.2
Alcohol	91.5	14.1	15.4
Cannabis	46.3	4.2	9.1

*Weighted estimates from the National Comorbidity Survey data gathered in 1990-1992 for persons 15-54 years old (n=8,098).

Adapted from: Anthony JC, Warner LA, Kessler RC. Comparative epidemiology of dependence on tobacco, alcohol, controlled substances, and inhalants: basic findings from the National Comorbidity Survey. Exp Clin Psychopharmacol 1994;2:244-268.

This overview is not intended to be comprehensive but is aimed at increasing the clinician's ability to recognize and better understand the clinical manifestations of addictive disease. The variations in the ways different individuals metabolize drugs from a neurobiologic standpoint could help explain why opioid treatment works well in some patients and causes problems in others.

Exposure Does Not Equal Addiction

It is a myth that everyone who takes opioids for chronic pain becomes addicted to the medication. This mistaken view is common even among many physicians. True opiate addiction that results from long-term opioid therapy is relatively rare. It is also rare in the wider US population. Consider the example of Vietnam veterans who revealed a high prevalence of heroin abuse and a high degree of physical dependence during wartime. In 1 study, about one-third of those veterans had recreationally experimented with heroin while overseas.[2] At home, however, their use of heroin and other narcotics returned to prewar levels. The results of that study show that not every individual becomes addicted to opioids, even when exposed to the most addicting substances (Box).

The question of why some people become addicted and others under similar circumstances do not remains a central challenge in drug-abuse research. More studies of the factors that confer either vulnerability or protection are needed. The results of some neuroimaging and experimental studies have shown that the brain of a person who is addicted to an opioid is very different in appearance and function from the brain of a nonaddicted individual. One goal of current neuroscience research is to understand the cellular and molecular mechanisms that mediate the transition from occasional controlled drug use to loss of behavioral control over drug seeking and drug taking (ie, addiction). To understand that transition, one must begin by examining the neuroanatomic involvement that is triggered when a person ingests an opioid medication.

Neuroanatomy

Addiction is a disease of the central nervous system. All substances of abuse activate essentially the same neuroanatomic structures that communicate by means of circuitry among structures. It is useful to have a global view of the major structures associated with addiction and to discuss their contributions. Each structure serves important purposes in daily life, but when that structure is exposed to substances of abuse, its functions are disturbed and undesirable consequences result.

As with most human behaviors, the behaviors associated with addiction are mediated by various inputs and outputs from multiple sites that function simultaneously. The entire central nervous system is involved with the disease of addiction, but certain structures more than others contribute to that state. A discussion of the major neurologic structures, their principal functions in a healthy individual, and how they react to chronic substance abuse follows.

Forebrain

The forebrain, which is the anterior and largest portion of the brain, contains the cerebral hemispheres and the limbic system. Each hemisphere is divided into 4 lobes: frontal, parietal, occipital, and temporal (Figure II:1). The forebrain controls cognitive, sensory, and

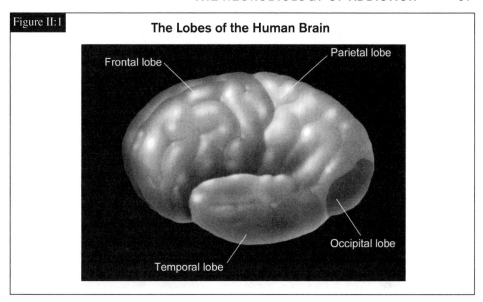

Figure II:1

The Lobes of the Human Brain

Frontal lobe

Parietal lobe

Occipital lobe

Temporal lobe

motor function and regulates temperature, reproductive functions, eating, sleeping, and the display of emotions. Chronic exposure to opioids and other substances of abuse may impact many of those functions.

Limbic System

The limbic system, which is contained within the forebrain, is composed of the limbic cortex and numerous subcortical structures. The euphoria experienced by drug abusers is caused by the stimulation of structures within the limbic system. The same structures are responsible for some of the primitive drives related to sex and eating. Neuroanatomists differ in opinion about what is considered a subcortical limbic structure of importance to the development of addiction. Regardless, it is generally agreed that the following structures are among the most important in that regard (Figure II:2):

- Frontal cortex.
- Prefrontal cortex.
- Anterior cingulate cortex.
- Hippocampal formation.
- Amygdala.
- Medial forebrain bundle.
- Nucleus accumbens.
- Nucleus locus ceruleus.
- Ventral palladium.
- Ventral tegmental area.

The limbic system monitors internal homeostasis and has a primary role in memory, learning, and emotion. Mega and colleagues described 2 divisions of the limbic system: an orbitofrontal-amygdala division, which is involved in emotional associations and appetites,

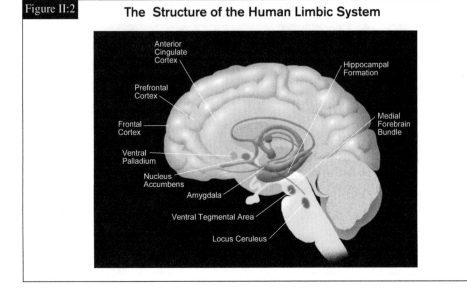

Figure II:2   The Structure of the Human Limbic System

and a hippocampus-cingulate division, which is involved with memory and attention.[3]

Abnormalities of the limbic structures correlate with disorders of emotion, mood, and thought. Positron emission tomography studies show increased activation in the limbic and paralimbic structures of patients experiencing drug craving.[4] In addition, these structures may also help mediate recurrent drug abuse.

Frontal Cortex

The frontal cortex receives sensory and emotional input from other sources in the brain and translates that input into behavior. For this reason, the frontal cortex is often known as the brain's "executive." Because the frontal cortex is so involved with evaluating events and planning complex cognitive and social behaviors, patients with dysfunction or lesions in that region of the brain will often display inappropriate behaviors and lack of insight.

Because of the diverse functions of the frontal cortex and its extensive interconnections with other nervous system structures, the behavioral syndromes caused by lesions of the frontal lobe may differ according to the location and size of the lesions. Damage to the frontal cortex can result in memory loss, disintegration of personality and emotional functioning, difficulty planning or initiating activity, severe apathy or euphoria, and a reduced ability to control thoughts, speech, or actions.

Similar deficits are believed to cause the bad decisions often made by people experiencing drug addiction. Recently, it has been shown that drug addiction is associated with functional changes in the frontal cortex that can lead to altered cognition and impaired inhibition of harmful behaviors.[5] It is also possible that such dysfunction predates and influences the substance abuse. With continued chronic drug exposure, the "executive functioning" of the frontal cortex becomes downregulated, and a less critical review of decision making results. This dysfunction is part of a syndrome called *impaired response inhibition and salience attribution*, in which conditioned cues to drug abuse become automatic and crowd out other rewarding stimuli.[5] It is possible (though unproven) that long-term opioid therapy can induce some of the changes in the frontal cortex that occur in patients with the disease of addiction.

Prefrontal Cortex

The frontal cortex can be divided into 3 major domains: precentral, limbic, and prefrontal. Of those 3 sections, the largest is the prefrontal cortex, which constantly updates the individual on the state of the environment. The prefrontal cortex is thought to help plan complex cognitive behaviors that express personality and social behavior. Impaired function of the prefrontal cortex is associated with immature judgment, impulsivity, and personality changes. The prefrontal cortex is not fully developed until a person reaches his or her early 20s. The immature judgment of adolescents may help to explain why the prevalence of drug abuse is higher in that age group than in other age groups.

Many older people with an addiction to opioids or other substances also display poor judgment and impulsivity. There is an association between long-term opioid dependence and cognitive and behavioral impairment that could be due in part to dysfunction of the prefrontal cortex. Personality changes are common in patients who abuse many drugs, and addicted people exhibit compulsive drug seeking that is fueled by an inability to make good decisions or to anticipate the consequences of poor decision making.[6] These cognitive problems are linked to deficits within the prefrontal cortex in some individuals before the first drug exposure, and it is likely that the function of the prefrontal cortex becomes compromised by repeated exposure to certain drugs.

Anterior Cingulate Cortex

The anterior cingulate cortex is a functional part of the limbic system that is active in cognitive and emotional tasks such as reward anticipation, decision making, and empathy. It also plays an important role in a wide variety of autonomic functions, including regulation of heart rate and blood pressure. Changes in the anterior cingulate cortex can be identified by means of neuroimaging equipment. Elevated activity in that anatomic region is associated with tics and obsessive-compulsive behavior. Conversely, reduced cingulate activity can contribute to diminished self-awareness, depression, and motor neglect.

The reward-anticipation function is important in opioid overconsumption. Neuroscientists believe that this area of the brain acts to encode reward values that lead to changes in behaviors based on the seeking of reward. People who are addicted become sensitized to environmental cues that are associated with pleasurable experiences, such as those that can be induced by opioids. When such cues are identified, the anticipation of reward is triggered, and drug-seeking behavior results.

Hippocampus and Hippocampal Formation

The hippocampus, which is inside the temporal lobe, mediates many functions, some of which are still poorly understood. Most neuroscientists agree that the hippocampus is instrumental in the formation of new episodic memories involving personal experiences. Others suggest that the hippocampus is responsible in part for mediating general memories, such as those involving facts. Over time and with the help of other brain structures, temporary memory is converted to long-term memory.

In addition to helping form new memories, the hippocampal formation is believed to be instrumental in the function of declarative memory that is associated with space and time. An example of this activity would be remembering the location of a supply of drugs or a rendezvous location for a drug pickup. The memory-creating functions of this anatomic area are thought to be a factor in repetitive pleasure-seeking behavior. The reinforcement of drug-seeking behavior requires that the brain recall a positive experience associated with drug use, and the pleasurable memory in turn produces a desire to repeat the drug-seeking behavior.

Damage to the hippocampus usually causes extreme difficulty in forming new memories. Although chronic stress has been shown to damage the hippocampus, it is unclear whether the chronic stress associated with pain and addiction is also linked to hippocampal damage and therefore to memory problems. Experts in the fields of addiction and pain management, however, observe that memory difficulties are common among substance abusers and chronic-pain patients.

Amygdala

Located deep within the temporal lobe, the amygdala appears critical in mediating drug craving and the recurrence of drug abuse. Its name reflects its distinctive heart shape, which is appropriate considering its place at the heart of many emotional processes. The functions of the amygdala include mediating the "fight or flight" response and the regulation of anxiety, fear, anger, and other emotions. It is important for feeling these emotions in oneself and for perceiving them in others. Because of those functions, the amygdala is the focus of much research into the evaluation of mood and emotion. The size and blood flow of the amygdala increase in people experiencing extraordinary emotional cues, such as those that occur during depression, and in people with posttraumatic stress disorder or bipolar disorder. In humans, stimulation of the amygdala produces fear, confusion, amnesia, and altered awareness. Anxiety and phobias may have their beginning in the abnormal functioning of this part of the brain. The amygdala is also involved in the modulation of food intake. Damage to certain areas of the amygdala induces hyperphagia, and stimulation can decrease appetite and arrest feeding behavior.

After the experience of drug abuse has been encoded, sensory and emotional stimuli can trigger a recurrence of drug-seeking behavior by re-evoking the reward experience. The hippocampal-amygdala complex receives that information and relates it to past events, particularly those associated with sights and smells.

The central role of the amygdala in modulating anxiety and fear may help explain the reasons some chronic-pain patients overuse opioids. After a patient has experienced severe pain, that sensation becomes part of his or her memory and can evoke anxiety in anticipation of another painful event. This aversive recall is processed through the hippocampal-amygdala complex and may explain why the anxiolytic effect of opioids appears to mollify some of the anxiety of anticipated pain. The desired anxiolytic effect can lead to the overuse of analgesics (a motivation unrelated to the seeking of euphoria).

Nucleus Accumbens

The nucleus accumbens, which is the brain's reward center, is always of prime importance in any discussion of the neuroanatomy of patients with an addiction. This area is flooded with "feel-good" chemicals (particularly the neurotransmitter dopamine) during drug use, and that pleasant sensation greatly reinforces drug-seeking behavior. For that reason, dopamine projections are essential to experiencing the rewarding properties of drugs.[7]

We have seen how the anterior cingulate cortex facilitates the anticipation of reward and the amygdala helps to process the stimuli associated with that reward. The nucleus accumbens contributes by mediating the motivation to behaviors associated with incentive.

Anterior Cingulate Gyrus ➤ Anticipated Reward
Amygdala ➤ Emotions
Nucleus Accumbens ➤ Motivation

The neurons of the nucleus accumbens communicate with the ventral palladium, which in turn sends the message along the reward pathway to the prefrontal cortex by means of dopamine transmission. The dopamine transmission to the structures of the forebrain originates in the ventral tegmental area, which is near the base of the brain. In addition to the nucleus accumbens, the ventral tegmental area is of central importance in understanding how messages are transmitted along the reward pathway. More detail on these chemical processes and circuitry will follow later in this chapter.

Nucleus Locus Ceruleus
The nucleus locus ceruleus is located in the brainstem. It is connected to the periaqueductal gray area, then to the nucleus accumbens, and then to the frontal cortex. Its extensive connective network gives the nucleus locus ceruleus the ability to integrate the functional activity of multiple brain regions. The nucleus locus ceruleus is involved in the response to stress and is believed to initiate rapid eye movement sleep. Stimulation of the locus ceruleus results in greater arousal, attention, and anxiety.

Locus Ceruleus ➤ Stress Response

When environmental stress and pain occur, the locus ceruleus expands with a greater density of neurons that stimulate, transmit, or receive the neurotransmitter norepinephrine. In a similar fashion, opioid withdrawal induces hyperactivity in this area via the stimulation of the sympathetic nervous system, which in turn results in the typical symptoms of abstinence syndrome (mydriasis, sweating, diarrhea, abdominal cramping).

It is believed that the release of norepinephrine from the locus ceruleus in the hippocampus enhances memory and facilitates the transition of new memory to long-term memory. The use of some illegal stimulants may mimic locus ceruleus stimulation and may contribute to the enhanced memory that is associated with the use of these drugs.

All of these structures of the brain are connected to the reward pathway of the central nervous system. However, no one brain region is responsible for the development of addiction. The amygdala is key to helping an organism determine whether or not to repeat an activity. The hippocampus records memories, including associations with environmental and other cues. Then, based on that input, the executive functions of the frontal cortex direct behavior. The reward pathway from the ventral tegmental area to the nucleus accumbens is influenced by the ingestion of drugs or other substances and is also associated with the memories and emotions that influence an individual's future choices to pursue rewarding stimuli.

Figure II:3 | Neurocircuitry of the Reward Pathway in the Human Brain

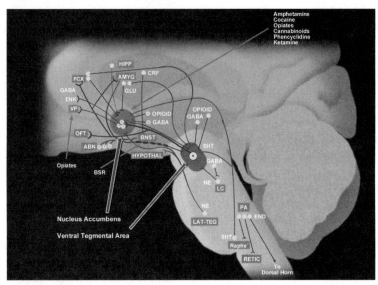

The mesolimbic dopamine system originates in the ventral tegmental area. Cell bodies project to the nucleus accumbens, the amygdala (AMYG), and the prefrontal cortex. Gamma-amino butyric acid (GABA), norepinephrine (NE), glutamatergic (GLU), and serotonergic (5-HT) projections are also important connections in the reward system of the human brain. The structures involved include the locus ceruleus (LC), hypothalamus (HYPOTHAL), lateral tegmental area (LAT-TEG), olfactory-frontal tract (OFT), ventral palladium (VP), and frontal cortex (FCX). The raphe nucleus has projections to the nucleus accumbens.

Neurocircuitry

To produce the drives and physiologic responses associated with addiction, it is necessary that the chief structures of the central nervous system communicate with each other and with other parts of the brain. This intercommunication is carried out via a complex circuitry of neurons (Figure II:3).

The ways in which the circuitry works have not been established, but recent evidence suggests that the mesolimbic dopaminergic system is the principal site at which drugs of abuse exert their power.[8] This region of the brain is linked to basic emotions and instincts. The main connection occurs through the medial forebrain bundle, which works like a power line of firing neurons and is sometimes called the "pleasure pathway" or the "reward pathway" (Figure II:4). To impart euphoria, all drugs of abuse must pass this way.[9]

The neuronal messages leading to euphoria and other drug effects travel by means of neurotransmitters, and the effect of dopamine is essential to understanding addictive processes. Dopamine projections originate in the ventral tegmental area and terminate in the amygdala, nucleus accumbens, prefrontal cortex, and ventral palladium. The dopamine pathway from the ventral tegmental area to the nucleus accumbens is so crucial to addiction that animals with lesions in that area stop seeking drugs of abuse.

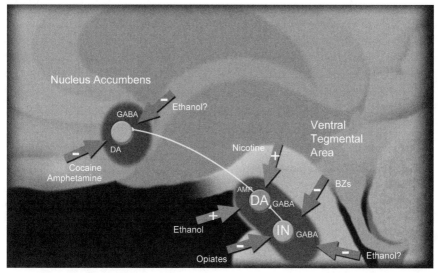

Figure II:4

Common Reward Pathway in the Human Brain

All substances of abuse use a common reward pathway. This schematic illustrates the sites at which the major substances of abuse impact the central nervous system. At the ventral tegmental area, many substances of abuse (BZs; benzodiazepines) can stimulate (+) or inhibit (-) the balance of dopamine (DA) and gamma-amino butyric acid (GABA) output.

The latest hypothesis of addiction suggests that the pleasure pathways of an addicted person are malfunctioning, probably because of disorders in brain chemistry, although scientists still lack a complete understanding of the precise mechanisms of the malfunction. Drug cravings can even be artificially induced by electrical stimulation of the brain. Experts have pointed out that the sites of the brain that are implicated in addiction are located not in the cerebral cortex, which mediates rational thought, but deep in the tissues that moderate instinctual drive.[10] For that reason, an addicted person cannot simply think his or her way out of addiction.

Addictive drugs exert a powerful influence over behavior, the result of the activation of brain circuitry. That power likely stems from the inability of the brain to differentiate the activation caused by drug intake from that related to eating, reproduction, and other activities necessary for survival. Any activity that triggers this same circuitry tends to be repeated, but the reward incentive delivered by addictive drugs is among the most powerful of stimuli.[11] The drive behind addiction is as commanding as the human instinct for survival.

Neurochemical Processes
Neurotransmitters

Dopamine is a neurotransmitter that exerts a powerful effect on emotion, including the capacity to experience pleasure or pain. Optimal levels of dopamine are critical to human health and well-being. People with Parkinson's disease have very little dopamine in their brain, and the delusions and hallucinations often experienced by people with schizophrenia result from too much dopamine.[7]

Dopamine has a leading role in all reinforcing behaviors. Food, drugs, and sex stimulate the delivery of dopamine or dopamine-mimicking effects from the ventral tegmental area to the nucleus accumbens. Addictive drugs cause a several-fold increase in the dopamine level of the nucleus accumbens. Indeed, the flooding of the nucleus accumbens by dopamine accounts for many of the primal pleasurable experiences known to humans. The resulting euphoria reinforces drug use but is not sufficient in itself to cause addiction. Conversely, a decrease in the dopamine level in the amygdala and the hippocampus may contribute to the anxiety and cravings that are often experienced by people with abstinence syndrome when drug use is stopped.

Opioids produce "rewards" via 2 basic mechanisms:
- They activate the ventral tegmental area and release dopamine in the nucleus accumbens.
- They bind directly to opiate receptors in the nucleus accumbens.

Dopamine has been called "the master molecule of addiction," but the story of how addiction develops is multifactorial, and other chemicals also contribute. Besides dopamine, other neurotransmitters linked to development of addiction include serotonin, norepinephrine, acetylcholine, glutamate, and gamma-amino butyric acid (GABA).

Glutamate and GABA are amino acids that act as major neurotransmitters in the central nervous system. Glutamate excites neurons, and GABA inhibits them. When opioids or

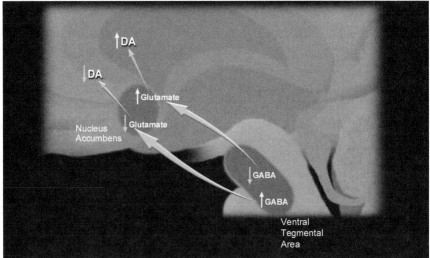

Figure II:5   **Alteration of the Reward Pathway for Glutamate and Gamma-Amino Butyric Acid**

An increase in gamma-amino butyric acid (GABA) at the ventral tegmental area decreases glutamate at the nucleus accumbens. This decreases the amount of dopamine (DA) released at the nucleus accumbens. Opioid stimulation of the ventral tegmental area inhibits GABA, which increases glutamate release at the nucleus accumbens. This results in an increase in DA.

other drugs are ingested, it is the decreased activity of GABA-inhibitory interneurons in the ventral tegmental area that causes the release of dopamine (Figure II:5). Glutamate activity appears to alter the reward pathway, reinforce memories of pleasant drug-engendered experiences, and cause the person to crave the same experience again. This occurs through a reduction in glutamate-mediated communication between cells in the nucleus accumbens.

Glutamate and GABA are present throughout the brain, and they use a greater number of synapses than do all other types of neurotransmitters combined. The widespread presence of GABA and glutamate presents a special challenge for creating addiction therapies that block the unwanted actions of drugs without producing adverse effects.

Opioid Receptors

Opioid receptors, which are located both inside and peripheral to the central nervous system, demonstrate widespread involvement in mood, affect, learning, memory acquisition, and many other physiologic functions. Opioids exert an analgesic effect by binding to opioid receptors, thereby blocking the transmission of pain signals. They cause euphoria by stimulating the regions of the brain that mediate pleasure. The structures and pathways that mediate addictive processes are also activated in the processing of pain control.

Opioids are known to bind to 3 receptor subtypes: mu, kappa, and delta. Mu and delta receptor subtypes, both of which are present in the ventral tegmental area and nucleus accumbens, exert power in opiate reinforcement. In contrast, activation of the kappa receptors can decrease dopamine release in the nucleus accumbens; thus, the kappa receptors do not produce a reward effect and may produce aversive responses.

Most opiates, including morphine, heroin, and methadone, are pure agonists at the mu receptor. Mu receptors mediate both the rewarding aspects of drugs and the development of physical dependence. It is interesting that knockout mice lacking mu-opioid receptors do not become physically dependent when given opioids.[6]

The greater release of dopamine from opioids into the nucleus accumbens is due to the high density of opioid receptors involved in the release of GABA in the ventral tegmental area. Stimulation of these receptors inhibits the release of GABA, thereby preventing its inhibitory effect and increasing the firing frequency of the dopamine neurons.[6]

Neuroadaptive Changes of Addiction

When the brain is exposed to an addictive drug, it begins immediately to adapt at a molecular level, which results in tolerance and sensitization.[12] It is clear that the "rush" from dopamine provides a major reinforcement in the continued abuse of drugs. However, the chemical effect of drug abuse does more than induce euphoria. After the stimulus is released, a learning process that "remembers" the euphoric, anxiolytic, or other positive effects of drug use occurs in the nervous system.

Learning and Neuroplasticity

According to the *Principles of Drug Addiction Treatment* published by the National Institute on Drug Abuse (NIDA), a brain repeatedly exposed to long-term substance abuse exhibits lasting changes (Figure II:6).[13] Those changes, which are both structural and functional, create in the vulnerable individual a behavioral compulsion to use drugs. As revealed by functional magnetic resonance imaging or positron emission tomography scanning, peo-

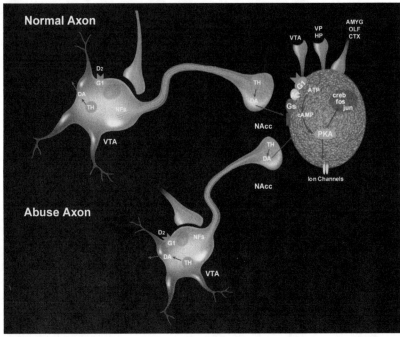

Figure II:6

Axons of Normal and Opioid Abuser States

The projection from the ventral tegmental area (VTA) to the nucleus accumbens (NAcc) changes over time after continued opioid exposure or in patients who are genetically predisposed to the disease of addiction. The left VTA neuron shows a robust connection to the NAcc neuron, and the stimulus of the NAcc has normal structure and function. The right VTA neuron illustrates the effects of long-term opioid exposure or opioid addiction in an individual who is genetically vulnerable to the disease of addiction. The connection to the NAcc on the right shows less structure and function than that of a healthy VTA neuron. This in turn affects the function of the NAcc.

ple addicted to cocaine show increased neuronal activity in the nucleus accumbens, even after merely having watched a video of someone else using the drug.[14] Among other effects, long-term drug abuse causes:

- Sensitization or heightened reward that changes gene expression in the mesolimbic dopamine system.
- Alterations in how glutamate and dopamine are transmitted in the nucleus accumbens.
- Changes in the neuronal structure throughout the pleasure pathway.

Chronic drug abuse impacts neuroplasticity, which is the basis of learning in the brain. The alteration of brain systems at the neural level is systematically demonstrated in behavior. The roles of memory and learning in addiction are relatively new areas of research. Decision-making capacities are not merely impaired in the addicted person; the decision-making apparatus is also damaged.

Tolerance

Tolerance to various effects produced by opioids tends to develop quickly. Tolerance to analgesia, for instance, requires that adequate pain relief be maintained via titration of doses or rotation to other opioids. In an abuse scenario, the more often a person takes a drug, the more drug he or she needs to achieve the level of pleasure (hedonia) formerly produced by the usual dosage. In the disease of addiction, gene-regulating activity dampens the brain's reward system by stimulating the production of chemicals that increase tolerance and decrease hedonia. This produces long-term set-point changes and modifications in gene expression. In other words, the person's hedonic set point is reset via the changes brought about by the constant bombardment of the nervous system with substances of abuse (Figure II:7).[15]

One of the several mechanisms that underlie tolerance can be explained by the fact that opioid receptors are known to be G-protein–coupled receptors. Repeated exposure to opioids uncouples the G protein and converts it from an inhibitory to an excitatory receptor. As the receptor becomes excitatory, a cascade of altered intracellular processes occurs that contributes to tolerance (Figure II:8). One intracellular mechanism underlying tolerance involves the cAMP response element-binding protein. Other intracellular changes include the production of intracellular free radicals that are toxic to the cells and contribute to the need for increased levels of opioid to produce the same effect. Soon, the addicted user needs more of the drug just to feel normal, even in the absence of liking the drug anymore. The

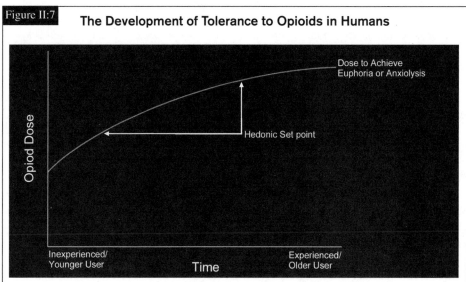

Figure II:7 **The Development of Tolerance to Opioids in Humans**

Opiod Dose

Dose to Achieve
Euphoria or Anxiolysis

Hedonic Set point

Inexperienced/
Younger User

Time

Experienced/
Older User

Over time, the dose of opioid required to produce the same euphoric or anxiolytic effect must be increased. This effect is defined as an increase in tolerance and a change in the hedonic set point.

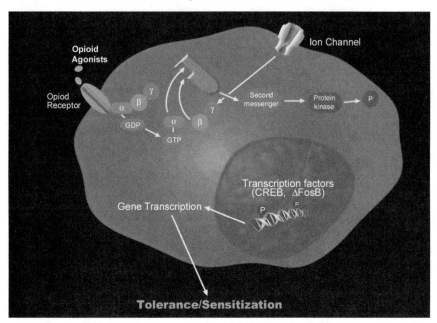

Figure II:8

The Molecular Activity of Tolerance and Sensitization

The neuroadaptation to long-term opioid exposure can lead to tolerance and sensitization. The molecular mechanisms involve initial stimulation of the opioid receptor, which inhibits intracellular transmission. Over time, the G-coupled proteins become uncoupled. The uncoupling of the G-proteins increases second messengers in protein kinase. Increases in protein kinase produce changes in the cAMP responsive element-binding protein (CREB) and FosB; this may lead to gene expression that could contribute to tolerance and sensitization.

rush produced by the drug is gone, but the compulsion to consume it persists and is coupled with a powerful craving that is divorced from any true reward. Even when harm occurs to health, relationships, and finances, the drug abuser cannot stop.

Sensitization

A person exposed and reexposed to a substance can become hypersensitive to its effects. When this occurs, the effects of the drugs are amplified. Sensitization lasts longer than tolerance induced by the cAMP response element-binding protein. It contributes to neuroplasticity and is likely the driving force behind the recurrence of abuse.

Behavioral sensitization stems from the cellular changes that involve learning and memory. The protein delta FosB is believed to be a factor in behavioral sensitization. High levels of this protein in the nucleus accumbens have been associated with hypersensitivity to drugs. During abstention from drug use, changes in both glutamate and delta FosB activity appear to foster sensitization, memories of the drug experience, and craving.[14] Drug-induced behavioral sensitization has been modeled in animals after repeated drug administration.[16-17]

Long-term drug abuse has also been shown to stimulate the growth of dendrite spines on neurons in the nucleus accumbens, thus likely boosting the neurons' signal-receiving capacities.[14] This early research could be a breakthrough in untangling the neuronal changes wrought by drug taking and may explain why those changes persist for so long. These changes to the nervous system mean that the addicted person "needs" the drug either to reinforce euphoria or to stop the negative consequences of abstinence syndrome or dysphoria. It is likely that many more mechanisms and chemicals are involved in the phenomenon of addiction, and it is difficult even to grasp the complexity of the addictive process. Each pathway or protein that is found to play a central role in addictive behaviors becomes another potential research target in the search for agents and treatments to prevent addiction.

Other Factors of Addiction
First Drug Exposure

For a vulnerable individual to manifest the disease of addiction, there must first be exposure to a psychogenic substance. In the case of opioid abuse, pharmacokinetics drives both the choice of the drug and the individual response to it. Abusers usually prefer the quick, intense high delivered by potent drugs with a rapid onset of action. Liposolubility facilitates the passage of a substance across the blood-brain barrier. Heroin is far more lipophilic than morphine, for example.

Genetics

Individual genetic variations greatly influence the effect of a drug on the patient, and this must be remembered when drugs are titrated to provide analgesia or other benefits. For example, variations in enzyme production in different individuals influence the rate at which codeine is metabolized to morphine. It is thus reasonable that the same types of differences also influence how people experience drug reward. The individual variations in the processing of pain, analgesia, and euphoria may all be genetically determined. This would explain why the disruption in brain function wrought by drug abuse feels negative to some people and pleasant or reassuring to others. A couple of findings contained in genetic research show that:

- Single-nucleotide polymorphisms (SNPs) of the gene that encodes the mu-opioid receptor are linked to an increased risk for heroin abuse. The most commonly occurring of these SNPs, A118G, results in a 3-fold increase in an endogenous opioid peptide.[18]
- The minor (A1) allele of the TaqIA D2 dopamine receptor gene is linked to severe alcoholism, polysubstance abuse, and opioid dependence.[19]

At least part of the vulnerability to addiction may stem from an individual's deficits in certain naturally occurring chemicals. Nearly 50 neurotransmitters have been shown to have an essential role in the development of addiction, and it is very possible that a chemical deficiency increases the vulnerability to addiction.[20] A person's direct or indirect ability to process dopamine may differ because of gene variations. This theory is supported by the results of research involving dopamine receptors, genes, and inhibitory enzymes that have yielded the hope of treatment to reduce the craving for nicotine and cocaine.

Cells do adapt to drug exposure by exhibiting long-term changes, but the disease of addiction is not activated in every individual. Although an initial exposure to a substance is needed to set the process of addiction in motion, some individuals have neurochemical, biological, and genetic vulnerabilities to addiction. They do not "choose" to become addicted, and their morals and strength of character are not necessarily less rigorous than those of people who do not become addicted when exposed to the same substance.

Environment

The most recent understanding of addiction, while acknowledging the powerful contribution of neurobiology, also accepts the need for specific environmental circumstances for full-blown addiction to occur. According to that perspective, addicted individuals are not labeled morally flawed characters, but neither are they viewed as helpless pawns.

People often wonder aloud why 1 child will grow up to exhibit the symptoms of addictive disease and others raised in the same family environment will not. The answer, of course, is that no 2 children, other than identical twins, are born with the same genetic makeup. Studies in which genetic factors correlate statistically with the likelihood of substance abuse by twins make this clear.[21] In addition, no 2 upbringings are identical, no matter how close in age the children are. Birth order, differences in parental expectations and directives, experiences with peers and other siblings, and individual responses to stresses of many types contribute their effects. The consequences for the individual are not superficial but profound.

Today's definition of addiction incorporates:
- Psychologic issues (eg, impaired control is an obsessive-compulsive preoccupation with the drug).
- Physical issues that address the primary loss of control as a neurochemical dysfunction.

The product created by the merging of these schools of thought is the biopsychosocial model of addiction. This is the model most frequently advanced in the scientific literature today.

Recurrence of Addiction

The evidence is strong that addiction is a neurobiologic disease rooted in individual genetic vulnerabilities. However, its expression is strongly influenced by psychosocial factors. Nowhere is this more true than when abuse recurs after a period of abstinence. A particular feature of addicted persons is their repeated return to drug use after having successfully cleansed their systems of the drug.

Much of what is known about the recurrence of addiction has been derived from animal models. Laboratory rats learn to self-administer the same drugs favored by human abusers, and environmental stress increases their self-administration of those agents. Some will choose the drug over food and sleep, even to the point of dying from malnutrition. They also demonstrate place preference for the environment in which the drug has been available in the past. The animals can then be kept "clean" for months, but they return to their prior drug-seeking behavior as soon as the substance is reinstated. The reward system of the animal brain "remembers" the drug.[14]

In 1 study, addicted rats displayed 3 diagnostic characteristics after having received a steady diet of cocaine for 3 months followed by abrupt termination of the drug.[22] They were persistent in trying to obtain the drug, they worked hard to get it, and they did not cease trying to obtain it, even when their feet were shocked during their efforts. As in humans, only a few rats (17%) displayed all 3 addictive criteria. Those that did were far more likely to experience a recurrence of addiction after a period of abstinence.

In humans, strong drug craving and the recurrence of addiction are most often precipitated by environmental factors:
- Reexposure to the drug (priming).
- Exposure to cues or stimuli previously paired with drug use.
- Stress.[8]

Priming, or a fresh exposure to a formerly abused substance, is an especially strong environmental cue to the recurrence of addiction. For a recovering person, it is also risky to be exposed to former drug-abusing peers, to enter situations (such as certain nightclubs or residences) in which abuse formerly occurred, or even to see the portrayal of a drug of choice being abused on television. Those events can stimulate intense craving in the addicted person who is trying to stay clear of the drug. Stress is also a strong factor in the recurrence of drug abuse. The stress that accompanies chronic pain, for example, can compel a recovering addicted person to resume active abuse.

Pain or Addiction: The Clinical Question

Euphoria and analgesia are mediated by the same mu receptors. Some of the drugs that are most effective in relieving pain also have the highest potential for being abused. The goal of opioid therapy is to reach an acceptable level of analgesia without triggering adverse effects such as excessive hedonia.

If the concept that addiction can coexist with chronic pain is accepted, then the clinical challenge is to discover which problem (pain or addiction) is primary. Fear of anticipated pain becomes strongly encoded in the memory of the chronic-pain patient. Opioids may have an anxiolytic effect that provides some patients with enough reinforcement to overuse their medication. Environment may be the factor that most often leads to opioid abuse in the chronic-pain population. The enormous stress related to inadequately treated pain coupled with low self-esteem and depression, which are common in patients experiencing chronic pain, may leave a patient vulnerable to the euphoric or obtunding effects of opioids. These effects may seem to provide an escape from harsh reality. In addition, physical tolerance can lead to the overuse of medication because the pain has become refractory to treatment with opioids.

Individuals display wide variations in the amount of opioids they require for pain relief or (in drug abusers) to obtain a high. The proclivity of an individual to develop compulsive use and craving for a substance varies in nearly infinite measure from another individual's tendency to do the same. Regardless of whether the abuse stems from addiction or some other cause, an estimated 6% to 15% of the US population has a serious substance-use disorder of some kind.[23] This can be seen as a threat to the integrity, safety, and efficacy of opioid therapy for pain.

To overfocus on determining whether patients are addicted could stigmatize certain patients and create a division among practitioners of different specialties. Perhaps a new category termed "opioid-related disorders" is needed. This nomenclature acknowledges that the range of substance-use disorders can be compared to the diversity of medical conditions that develop in patients with diabetes. One diabetic patient may exhibit relatively minor anomalies in insulin production, and another may have been born without insulin cells. Both, however, require treatment suited to their individual needs. Substance-use disorders also have many manifestations; universal absolutes do not apply. These interpatient variations must be acknowledged to achieve optimal treatment.

Participants in Narcotics Anonymous frequently say, "You're an addict when you say you are." It may be less important for clinicians to definitively establish whether patients are addicted than to ascertain whether their primary problem is uncontrolled pain or uncontrolled substance use and to tailor treatment accordingly.

Conclusion

According to common opinion, anyone exposed to opiates or other strong drugs at high enough doses for long enough will become addicted. The disease of addiction is now recognized as being far more complex than such a basic premise. Exposure to the drug must occur, but more than exposure is required for addiction to develop. Evidence strongly suggests that the development of addiction requires a predetermined genetic framework. The disease process then requires repeated exposures to a substance that produces a reward in the limbic system by increasing the availability of dopamine. Repeated drug consumption alters existing pathways by inducing tolerance and sensitization. This overstimulation leads to long-term or permanent changes in the secondary messengers that trigger craving, impaired control over drug use, compulsive drug use, and continued drug use despite harm. People who abuse drugs exhibit specific behaviors. The next chapter will examine the most common behaviors associated with problematic opioid use and the motivations that drive them.

References

1. Quotes by Shirley Chisholm. Answers.com Web site. Available at: http://www.answers.com/topic/shirley-chisholm. Accessed April 10, 2007/

2. Robins LN, Helzer JE, Davis DH. Narcotic use in southeast Asia and afterward. An interview study of 898 Vietnam returnees. Arch Gen Psychiatry. 1975 Aug;32(8):955-61.

3. Mega MS, Cummings JL, Salloway S, Malloy P. The limbic system: an anatomic, phylogenetic, and clinical perspective. J Neuropsychiatry Clin Neurosci. 1997 Summer;9(3):315-30.

4. Kilts CD, Schweitzer JB, Quinn CK, Gross RE, Faber TL, Muhammad F, Ely TD, Hoffman JM, Drexler KP. Neural activity related to drug craving in cocaine addiction. Arch Gen Psychiatry. 2001 Apr;58(4):334-41.

5. Goldstein RZ, Volkow ND. Drug addiction and its underlying neurobiological basis: neuroimaging evidence for the involvement of the frontal cortex. Am J Psychiatry. 2002 Oct;159(10):1642-52.

6. Cami J, Farre M. Drug addiction. N Engl J Med. 2003 Sep 4;349(10):975-86.

7. Joseph MH, Datla K, Young AM. The interpretation of the measurement of nucleus accumbens dopamine by in vivo dialysis: the kick, the craving or the cognition? Neurosci Biobehav Rev. 2003;27(6):527-41.

8. Bryant CD, Zaki PA, Carroll FI, Evans CJ. Opioids and addiction: Emerging pharmaceutical strategies for reducing reward and opponent processes. Clin Neurosci Res 2005; 5:103-15.

9. Gardner EL. Addictive potential of cannabinoids: the underlying neurobiology. Chem Phy Lipids. 2002 Dec 31;121(1-2):267-90.

10. The hijacked brain. Addiction Treatment Forum. Winter 2000;9(1):3-5. Available online at www.ATForum.com.

11. Gardner EL. What we have learned about addiction from animal models of drug self-administration. Am J Addict. 2000 Fall;9(4):285-313.

12. O'Brien CP, Gardner EL. Critical assessment of how to study addiction and its treatment: human and non-human animal models. Pharmacol Ther 2005 Oct;108(1):18-58.

13. National Institute on Drug Abuse, National Institutes of Health, US Department of Health and Human Services. Principles of drug addiction treatment: a research-based guide. NIH Publication No. 00-4180. Rockville, MD. Printed October 1999, Reprinted July 2000.

14. Nestler EJ, Malenka RC. The addicted brain. Scientific American; March 2004: 78-85.

15. Koob GF, Le Moal M. Drug abuse: hedonic homeostatic dysregulation. Science. 1997 Oct 3;278(5335):52-8.

16. Thomas MJ, Beurrier C, Bonci A, Malenka RC. Long-term depression in the nucleus accumbens: a neural correlate of behavioral sensitization to cocaine. Nat Neurosci. 2001 Dec;4(12):1217-23.

17. Brebner K, Wong TP, Liu L, Liu Y, Campsall P, Gray S, Phelps L, Phillips AG, Wang YT. Nucleus accumbens long-term depression and the expression of behavioral sensitization. Science 2005 Nov 25;310(5752):1340-3.

18. Kreek MJ. Pain management and chemical dependency: observations of a neuroscientist and clinician. 3rd International Conference on Pain Management and Chemical Dependency; New York, NY: Jan. 28-30, 1999.

19. Noble EP. D2 dopamine receptor gene in psychiatric and neurologic disorders and its phenotypes. Am J Med Genet B Neuropsychiatr Genet. 2003 Jan 1;116(1):103-25. Review.

20. Gardner EL. The neurobiology and genetics of addiction: implications of the "Reward Deficiency Syndrome" for therapeutic strategies in chemical dependency. In: Elster J, ed. *Addiction: Entries and Exits.* New York: Russell Sage Foundation;1999:57-119.

21. Kendler KS, Aggen SH, Tambs K, Reichborn-Kjennerud T. Illicit psychoactive substance use, abuse and dependence in a population-based sample of Norwegian twins. Psychol Med. 2006 Jul;36(7):955-62.

22. Deroche-Gamonet V, Belin D, Piazza PV. Evidence for addiction-like behavior in the rat. Science. 2004 Aug 13;305(5686):1014-7.

23. Passik SD, Kirsh KL. Managing pain in patients with aberrant drug-taking behaviors. J Support Oncol. 2005 Jan-Feb;3(1):83-6.

CHAPTER III

PATIENT BEHAVIOR AND OPIOID ABUSE

When you see misuse behavior, that's a question to be answered.
- Steven D. Passik, PhD, pain psychologist and palliative care specialist
(oral communication, March 2004)

No radiograph or diagnostic test can reveal whether a person is addicted to or abusing opioid medication. To date, a clinician's only available tools used to screen for detrimental drug use are the observation and interpretation of a patient's behavior. The difficulty of this task is illustrated by the following sentence in the text by Burglass and Shaffer:[1] "Certain individuals use certain substances in certain ways thought at certain times to be unacceptable by certain other individuals for reasons both certain and uncertain." The ambiguity of that statement represents a clinical challenge, because a patient's motivation for engaging in aberrant drug-related behavior may be influenced by a variety of conditions and circumstances of which addictive disease is only a part. If pain treatment with opioids is to be successful, prescription misuse must be managed. To accomplish this, it is necessary to monitor, document, and address a patient's aberrant drug-related behavior. The goal is to ensure that opioid therapy is beneficial to the patient rather than a source of unmanageable difficulty.

Types of Aberrant Drug-Related Behavior

Certain patient behaviors are commonly thought to indicate problems with managing opioid intake. In the broadest sense, an aberrant behavior is any drug-related deviation from the medical plan. Listed in no particular order of importance are some of these aberrant drug-related behaviors: [2-3]

- Unauthorized dose escalation on 1 occasion.
- Unauthorized dose escalation on more than 1 occasion.
- Prescription forgery.
- Selling prescriptions.
- Using opioids to achieve euphoria.
- Using opioids for relief of anxiety.
- Overdose.
- Injecting oral formulations.
- Abnormal results from urinalysis or blood screening.
- Soliciting opioids from multiple prescribers.
- Unauthorized emergency department visits.
- Concurrent abuse of alcohol, illegal drugs, or other prescribed medications.
- Resisting changes to therapy or the use of alternative therapies.
- Reporting lost or stolen prescriptions.
- Repeatedly canceling appointments.
- Requesting early refills.
- Requesting refills instead of an appointment with the physician.

- Being discharged from a clinician's practice for noncompliance.
- Not showing up for follow-up appointments.
- Altering the route of drug administration.
- Hoarding drugs.
- Purposeful oversedation.
- Appearing intoxicated.
- Insisting on treatment with a specific medication.
- Participating in street drug culture.
- Being arrested by police for drug-related activities.
- Having a vehicle accident or another accident related to drug use.

According to 3 medical associations that collaborated on a 2001 consensus document related to the use of opioids,[4] additional behaviors that should cause concern include:

Box III:1   **Behaviors Predictive of Drug Addiction**

Aberrant Behaviors Less Predictive of Addiction

- Aggressive complaining about need for a higher dose.
- Drug hoarding when symptoms are milder.
- Requesting specific drugs.
- Acquiring similar drugs from other medical sources.
- Unsanctioned dose escalation once or twice.
- Unapproved use of the drug to treat another symptom.
- Reporting psychiatric drug-related effects not intended by the clinician.
- Occasional impairment.

Aberrant Behaviors More Predictive of Addiction

- Selling prescription drugs.
- Prescription forgery.
- Stealing or "borrowing" drugs from another person.
- Injecting oral formulations.
- Obtaining prescription drugs from a nonmedical source.
- Multiple episodes of prescription "loss."
- Concurrent abuse of related illicit drugs.
- Multiple dose escalations despite warnings.
- Repeated episodes of gross impairment or dishevelment.

Source: Portenoy RK. Opioid therapy for chronic nonmalignant pain: a review of the critical issues. J Pain Symptom Manage. 1996 Apr;11(4):203-17.

- Isolation from family and friends.
- Insisting on rapid-onset formulations of prescribed drugs.
- Reporting no relief from any nonopioid treatment.
- Using analgesic medications for effects other than analgesia.

It is often difficult for clinicians to determine which type or frequency of behavior indicates the most serious drug abuse problems. Long-term prospective studies on that topic are scarce, but some behaviors are said to be more predictive and others less predictive of addiction (Box III:1). Most pain experts would probably agree that a patient who forges prescriptions or who crushes and ingests a tablet is engaging in more worrisome behavior than is a patient who occasionally takes an extra pill to relieve breakthrough pain. However, given the scarcity of empirical data, researchers and specialists in pain management have found little agreement on the concrete significance of many drug-related behaviors. This impasse is highlighted in a pilot study in which 100 pain-management physicians ranked common aberrant behaviors in order of severity (Box III:2).[5] Although the selling of prescriptions is listed first and the patient's unkempt appearance is deemed least important, every behavior appeared at least once in all 13 ranking slots over the course of the survey. Obviously, there is great variation in how physicians perceive the seriousness of the most common behaviors in their patients.

However, some progress in isolating the behaviors most associated with addictive disease has been made. A study by Compton and colleagues found the following 3 characteristics to be the most accurate identifiers of substance-dependent subjects:

Box III:2

Aberrant Drug-Related Behaviors

(From most aberrant to least aberrant behavior)
- Selling prescription drugs.
- Forging prescriptions.
- Altering the route of administration or the drug delivery system (eg, crushing controlled-release tablets for snorting or injection).
- Concurrent abuse of related illicit drugs.
- Stealing or borrowing medications from others.
- Obtaining drugs from a nonmedical source.
- Frequent loss of prescriptions.
- Multiple occasions of unsanctioned dosing.
- Aggressively demanding more drugs.
- Unapproved use of drugs to treat nonpainful symptoms.
- Drug hoarding.
- Unsanctioned dose escalation once or twice.
- Unkempt appearance.

Source: Passik SD, Kirsh KL, Whitcomb L, Dickerson PK, Theobald DE. Pain clinicians' rankings of aberrant drug-taking behaviors. J Pain Palliat Care Pharmacother. 2002;16(4):39-49.

- The tendency to increase analgesic dose or frequency.
- Requests for a preferred route of drug administration.
- Considering oneself addicted.[6]

That study also revealed strong family dynamics among addicted patients, including the sharing of medications and other enabling patterns.

Experts have joined together to attempt to define criteria for problematic drug use. A committee of pain providers created a 5-point checklist for use in monitoring the incidence of prescription opiate abuse in patients with chronic nonmalignant pain. The items deemed consistent with prescription opiate abuse are:

- An overwhelming, time-consuming focus on prescription opiates persisting beyond the third treatment session.
- A pattern of early prescription refills (3 or more) or an escalation of drug dose unexplained by a medical condition.
- Placing multiple phone calls to or otherwise creating a disturbance with office staff about prescription issues.
- A pattern of lost, spilled, or stolen prescriptions.
- Supplemental sources of opiates obtained from multiple providers, emergency departments, or illegal sources.[7]

In the end, the determination of whether a patient's behavior is detrimental and indicates a serious abuse problem is, by necessity, subjective. The clinician must exercise his or her medical judgment in making such determinations and must be guided by the best available evidence-based science and the consensus of experts in the field.

Prevalence and Significance of Aberrant Behavior

Compliance with opioid treatment is vital, but noncompliance is common. Aberrant behavior of any type, severity, or frequency interferes with the safe and effective delivery of pain relief via opioid therapy. If a patient uses a prescribed medication in ways that defy medical direction, the prescribing clinician cannot accurately assess the effects of that drug. For example, if a physician wrongly assumes that a drug has been used as directed and with that understanding makes an adjustment such as increasing or decreasing the dosage or adding an additional medication, the outcome could harm the patient. Taking too much of a prescribed medication or mixing it with other substances such as alcohol, illegal drugs, or other opioids could result in a toxic interaction. If a physician finds the patient untrustworthy and consequently prescribes less of an opioid than would normally be effective, the patient's pain may worsen and the outcome of treatment may be compromised.

Given the potential hazards, it is unfortunate that patient noncompliance with prescribed drug therapy is widespread. Recent studies suggest that there is a higher prevalence of aberrant behavior among pain patients treated with prescribed opioids than pain management experts had previously thought. Here are just a few examples from the scientific literature:

- A study conducted in the author's pain clinic found aberrant drug-related behavior in 40% of 185 chronic-pain patients who were monitored for 1 year.[2]

• Thirty-four percent of 76 chronic-pain patients receiving long-term prescription opiate therapy met at least 1 criterion for prescription drug abuse, and 28% met 3 or more of those criteria.[7]

• As evaluated by their own physicians, 45% of 388 patients with nonmalignant pain displayed at least 1 behavior suggestive of noncompliance during treatment.[8]

• A study of 109 chronic-pain patients found that 21% had concealed polymedication consumption, which was verified by urine screening, from their physicians.[9]

• Random urine samples failed to show the expected dose concentrations in 54% of 14,712 outpatient pain patients treated with sustained-release oxycodone.[10]

• Drug abuse behavior was recorded in 24% of patients treated in Veterans Administration medical facilities and in 31% of primary care patients in a retrospective study of 98 patients with chronic nonmalignant pain who were treated with opioids for 6 months or longer during a 1-year period.[11]

Those statistics are certainly sobering. However, to understand them in context, the clinician must realize that the presence of aberrant behaviors seldom denotes the presence of addictive disease. In fact, aberrant behaviors are not even synonymous with the definition of opioid abuse. A look at the various categories of abuse behavior will help to clarify those concepts.

"The Circles:" Relationships Among Aberrant Behavior, Abuse, and Addiction

About 1% of the general US population exhibits opioid addiction.[12] The prevalence of addiction among opioid-treated chronic-pain patients (2%-5%) in the first author's pain clinic is a little higher than that statistic (Figure III:1).[2] A much larger group (20%) is prone

---

Figure III:1   Aberrant Behavior, Abuse, and Addiction in a Pain Clinic

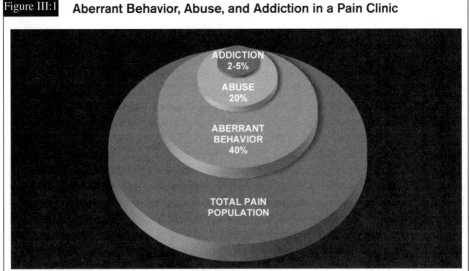

Source: *Webster LR, Webster RM. Predicting aberrant behaviors in opioid-treated patients: preliminary validation of the Opioid Risk Tool. Pain Med. 2005 Nov-Dec;6(6):432-42.*

to abuse. Still greater is the number of pain patients in the study who exhibit some form of aberrant behavior (approximately 40% display at least 1 such behavior). The circles in Figure III:1 demonstrate how seldom it is that aberrant behaviors can clearly be said to stem from addictive disease, which is characterized by uncontrolled drug use, craving for the drug, compulsion to use the drug, and continued drug use despite harm. Although some of the patients who fall into the "abuse" category may be revealed at a later date to be addicted to a drug, a fair number are not addicted but misuse their medication for other reasons. It would probably be accurate to say that all addicted people are abusers, but not all abusers are addicted.

Another striking point is that only half of the patients who display at least one aberrant behavior can be classified as abusers. A behavior is considered aberrant if it deviates from the accepted medical treatment plan; however, in clinical practice, true opioid abusers demonstrate more than 1 or 2 relatively minor aberrant behaviors. To grasp this point, consider the following example of a 1-time request for an early refill:

> A senior woman for whom 2 tablets of hydrocodone-acetaminophen per day were prescribed as treatment for arthritis pain instead used 4 tablets per day a few times during the month when greater pain relief was needed. Consequently, she ran out of her medication a few days early because she had overused it.

Though this behavior is by definition aberrant (like any other intentional overuse of medication), most physicians would not classify this minor deviation as opioid abuse. In most instances, drug abuse involves deception and the intent to use a drug for a nonmedical purpose or repeated infractions. Abuse in a clinical context is characterized by continued aberrant behaviors that, based on observation, appear to be making it difficult for the patient to cope. That is the point at which clinical knowledge and skill are needed. The judgment of when aberrant behavior becomes abuse is of necessity made by the clinician.

The Continuum of Abuse

The depiction of aberrant behaviors (Box III:1) as "more predictive" or "less predictive" of addiction can be oversimplified if it is interpreted too literally. The behaviors shown in the "less predictive" column of that Box can also occur when serious abuse is taking place, and it is difficult to classify specific behaviors as "red flags" that clearly indicate addiction or other severe problems.

It is probably clinically accurate to say that aberrant behaviors exist on a continuum ranging from none to egregious with an infinite number of positions between those 2 poles (Figure III:2). To the far left of the spectrum are the patients who keep appointments, take all their medications as directed, and act as advocates for their own welfare. To the far right are patients who engage in such obviously egregious behavior as crushing their pills and injecting them intravenously.

Patients who are addicted most often engage in multiple aberrant behaviors. Some pain-management specialists suspect that the number of aberrant behaviors displayed is more important than the type of behavior. In the first author's pain clinic, patients classified as being at high risk for opioid abuse or addiction demonstrated more than 4 times the number of aberrant behaviors than did those in the moderate-risk group.[1] Patients at high risk

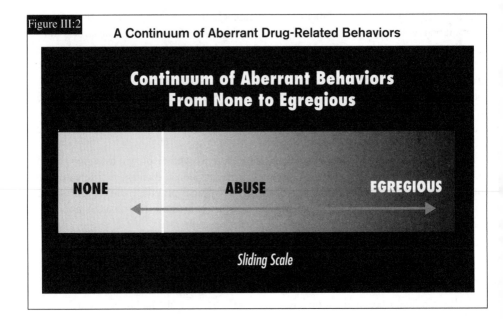

Figure III:2   **A Continuum of Aberrant Drug-Related Behaviors**

for addiction also tended to demonstrate aberrant behaviors sooner than did patients whose risk level was relatively lower.

However, even 1 egregious behavior, such as injecting oral formulations or forging prescriptions, can point to addiction or another serious difficulty with managing opioid intake. To further complicate matters, people do not necessarily occupy 1 point on the continuum of risk throughout their lifetimes; their status can change as a result of new circumstances or medical conditions, the substance or substances consumed, the advent of psychologic difficulties, etc.

Appropriate medical care, including that for people with addictive disease, depends on monitoring the patient's progress, pain relief, physical function, quality of life, and compliance with opioid therapy over time. Even if the patient's motivations for medication misuse are unclear, the right action is always to address any aberrant behaviors that appear.

Classifying Aberrant Behavior

It should be apparent by now that the classification of aberrant behaviors according to their significance is anything but an exact science. Most experts agree that exhibiting many types of aberrant behavior or demonstrating 1 or 2 egregious behaviors is likely to indicate trouble. However, few controlled studies have determined the importance of each aberrant behavior in pinpointing a substance-use disorder. That lack of certainty does not mean that clinicians cannot judge whether the success of opioid therapy is being threatened by aberrant behavior. To further this endeavor, serious attention should be paid to the characteristics of the aberrant behaviors being observed.

Classification by Characteristics of Abuse

Certain characteristics observed over time can help clinicians to gauge the depth of an individual's problems with managing opioid intake. These properties of aberrant behaviors include:

- *Their relative severity.* The presence of egregious behaviors (crushing and then injecting or snorting formulations, stealing medications, or forging prescriptions) indicates serious abuse and possible addiction.
- *Their quantity.* Multiple aberrant behaviors can be a sign that drug use is out of control. The more aberrant behaviors an individual exhibits, the more likely the individual is abusing or is addicted to opioids.
- *Their persistence.* Recurrent aberrant behavior despite repeated warnings can be considered abuse and may signify addiction.
- *Their purpose.* Patients with severe abuse problems deliberately misuse their medication for reasons of their own, such as addiction or another underlying cause.
- *Their time-consuming nature.* The more time and healthcare resources required to manage a patient's manifestations of aberrant behavior, the greater the cause for the suspicion of severe abuse.

Classification by Type of Abuse

It is true that aberrant behaviors cannot be classified strictly according to risk; the number and persistence of behaviors may be more important than the type of behavior in some patients. However, some single behaviors are considered more egregious and others could be considered lower risk, particularly if they do not recur. Perhaps it would be useful to examine some of the common behaviors and consider their possible causes. The following behaviors could be considered *low risk* if they are observed on 1 or 2 occasions but may be of greater concern if they recur or are manifested in a pattern of abuse in combination with other behaviors:

- *Reporting lost or stolen prescriptions.* A single occurrence of this behavior is common and could be due to an innocuous incident such as dropping pills down the sink. The behavior should be documented and watched for recurrence.
- *Unauthorized dose escalation.* One or 2 reports of this behavior are common, but the concern of abuse increases with repeated incidents. The patient should be counseled about the necessity of complying with treatment instructions.
- *Appointment cancelation.* This low-risk behavior could stem from several legitimate causes. As with all such behaviors, it should be documented to track whether it is repeated or is manifested in a pattern with other behaviors.
- *Requesting early refills.* Such a request may stem from a serious pain problem during which an extra dose of medication helped the patient to cope. The clinician should adjust the treatment plan. If the patient is still unable to comply, this behavior moves from a low-risk to a moderate-risk indicator.
- *Requesting refills instead of an appointment.* This behavior should be documented and monitored as a potential pattern but is considered low risk because it could stem from a legitimate issue.
- *Not showing up for follow-up appointments.* This relatively low-risk behavior could have a variety of meanings, including the possibility that the patient disliked the clinician's manner and sought care elsewhere.

The following *moderate-risk behaviors* require careful monitoring. Patients should receive firm compliance counseling, and the clinician should attempt to discern the underlying problem that is driving the behavior.

- *Unauthorized dose escalation on more than one occasion.* Repetition of this behavior increases concern. Lack of pain control should be suspected. If titration to an analgesic dose results in decreased functioning and continued escalations in the dose, the patient should be carefully evaluated for comorbid psychiatric disorders or addictive disease.
- *Using opioids to relieve anxiety.* This indicates an underlying anxiety disorder that needs treatment independent of pain therapy.
- *Abnormal results from a urine or blood screening.* This objective verification of noncompliance varies in significance depending on what the screening reveals. If, for example, cocaine or heroin is found, the classification of the behavior moves from "moderate" to "serious." The presence of tetrahydrocannabinol is also a problem, though a relatively milder one. The concomitant abuse of benzodiazepines may indicate the presence of an anxiety disorder. Absence of the expected quantities of opioids in the results of urine or blood screening could signify the criminal act of diverting medications for sale. It is important to note, document, and evaluate the variety and quantity of the substances found in the results of blood and urine screenings.
- *Soliciting opioids from other prescribers.* This moderate-to-high-risk behavior requires an element of deception on the part of the patient and should cause concern. Possible causes will be explored later in this text. A few of the possible reasons for the unauthorized seeking of additional doses could include undertreated or otherwise uncontrolled pain, active addiction, or criminal diversion.
- *Unauthorized emergency department visits.* It is important to examine the patient's real or perceived need for more medication, whether it is for legitimate pain relief or some other purpose. This behavior is deemed aberrant primarily if it causes inconvenience to the clinician. Some clinicians actually encourage patients to visit an emergency department as opposed to calling after hours. Other clinicians consider unauthorized emergency department visits grounds for dismissal.
- *Resisting changes in therapy or the use of alternative therapies.* A legitimate reason could exist, but a complete refusal to consider proven procedures should arouse concern.
- *Insisting on treatment only with a specific and named medication.* This behavior could suggest a problem, or it could result from the proven pain relief experienced by the individual after treatment with the prescribed drug. The indication is stronger if the specific drug demanded is a rapid-onset analgesic.
- *Having been discharged from another clinician's practice for noncompliance.* A moderate-to-high-risk indicator that tends to confirm some type of problem.

Some behaviors suggest *serious problems*, even if they are observed only once:

- *Prescription forgery.* This is a criminal offense. The clinician is obligated to dismiss the patient from care at the first occurrence.
- *Selling prescriptions.* This criminal offense also calls for the immediate dismissal of the patient.
- *Injecting oral formulations.* This serious behavior is likely to stem from addictive disease and to reflect compulsive drug use despite harm.
- *Overdose.* An overdose could originate from several causes, such as a provider error in prescribing or a patient error in consuming medication, a suicide attempt to escape unrelieved pain or overwhelming life stress, a psychiatric disorder, the overuse of or the combining of substances used for recreational purposes, or addictive disease.
- *Altering the route of administration.* Crushing or otherwise altering medications is a serious behavior that cannot be tolerated and must be addressed immediately. It is possible that the behavior could result from the desire to relieve uncontrolled pain or some other nonaddiction source, but it also demonstrates a street-savvy approach to medication that should cause concern.

The general alerts cited above were noted during years of clinical experience in observing and treating patients with chronic pain. Additional research should help to clarify the significance of abuse behaviors, but nothing will ever replace sound clinical judgment and the awareness of patients as individuals rather than clusters of symptoms. Every healthcare professional is called on to apply those standards every day.

Different Faces of Abuse
When clinicians observe the symptoms of aberrant drug-related behavior in their patients, they might instantly suspect an addictive disorder but could actually be treating a patient who has any of a variety of conditions, some of which are listed in Box III:3[13] and

---

Box III:3   Differential diagnosis of aberrant drug-related behavior

Addiction.
Pseudoaddiction (uncontrolled pain).
Other psychiatric disorders.
- Axis I disorders (eg, anxiety disorders, major depression).
- Axis II disorders (eg, personality disorders such as borderline personality, antisocial personality).
Encephalopathy associated with medication toxicity.
Psychosocial or emotional issues (eg, family discord, financial worries, work-related discontent, "rebellion").
Recreational use (eg, experimentation, pleasure, escape, peer pressure).
Criminal intent.

Source: Kirsh KL, Whitcomb LA, Donaghy K, Passik SD. Abuse and addiction issues in medically ill patients with pain: attempts at clarification of terms and empirical study. Clin J Pain. 2002 Jul-Aug;18(14 Suppl):S52-60.

Box III:4

It May Look Like Addiction: Other Reasons for Abuse

- *Uncontrolled pain (pseudoaddiction)*. Intentional medication misuse characterized by drug-seeking behavior that results from the significant undertreatment of pain.
- *Chemical coping*. Intentional misuse of medication as a result of psychologic stress or mental disease. The usual outcome is a decrease in function and quality of life.
- *Rational abuse*. Intentional misuse of medication; improves the patient's function and quality of life, whether the misuse arises from uncontrolled pain, an undiagnosed mental disorder, or another cause.

Box III:4. The patient's motive for aberrant behavior matters; that motive can reveal underlying problems such as substance abuse or a psychiatric disorder that requires treatment in addition to therapy to relieve pain.

Any intentional misuse of opioid medications (not just the compulsive consumption of the addicted person or the willful behavior of the recreational abuser) can be dangerous. For pain treatment to be successful, problems with abuse must be managed. This can only be accomplished by accurately isolating, diagnosing, and treating the separate problems that are driving the abuse.

When aberrant behavior is observed, perhaps the first diagnosis to consider should be that of uncontrolled pain. Referrals for psychiatric consultation or behavioral counseling can uncover the presence of mental disease, family stress, and other underlying factors. The possibility for frank criminal intent in obtaining drugs to sell will be discussed in a later chapter. Some aberrant behavior is the result of an active addiction in which pain may or may not also be present. The challenge is to determine the appropriate treatments, actions, or referrals that are based on the individual patient's profile.

Uncontrolled Pain ("Pseudoaddiction")

A patient may suffer from pain that is not controlled by prescribed medication. Perhaps that patient, for individual physiologic reasons, is unable to reach the therapeutic window at which pain relief occurs for most patients who receive opioid therapy, or perhaps the quantity of opioid prescribed is inadequate. The patient then escalates the dose or otherwise defies medical orders in an attempt to curb the pain.

The resulting drug-seeking behavior may look like addiction, but it is not. If the patient had not experienced pain or required treatment with opioids, a substance-abuse problem would not have developed. The patient may seek prescriptions from more than 1 provider or may repeatedly visit a hospital emergency department. He or she may even alter a prescription to obtain more medication. The term "uncontrolled pain patient" describes a patient whose pain and drug-seeking behavior are both out of control. That definition is preferable to the less precise though widely used term "pseudoaddict."[14] It is no surprise such patients are often labeled "drug seekers." Their clinical profiles closely resemble those of addicted patients. It is correct to say that the addicted patient's motive, at least initially, is to seek euphoria or other psychogenic rewards from opioids and that the motive of the patient with uncontrolled pain is to achieve adequate pain control. However, because both patients engage in similar aberrant behaviors, such as escalating doses without authorization, it can be difficult to differentiate between them. The difference, which may be revealed over time and with clinical observation, is this:

- The addicted patient loses function and quality of life after inappropriate drug use.
- The patient with uncontrolled pain gains function and quality of life after pain has been adequately controlled with appropriate therapy.

In theory, titrating the medication to an analgesic dose should expose the truth by removing the reason for drug-seeking behavior in the patient with uncontrolled pain. This is true in most cases and should be the clinician's first response. After the pain has been adequately controlled, the patient's focus on obtaining more opioids should become less intense, and the aberrant behavior should stop. Thus the patient with uncontrolled pain does not exhibit the drug craving, compulsion to obtain the drug, loss of control, or continued use of the drug despite harm, as do truly addicted patients. However, some pain, such as neuropathic pain, is often refractory to opioid treatment. If that occurs, the problem is not that giving opioids causes abuse, but that the pain is untreatable with currently available medications. That scenario can lead to unabated aberrant behaviors that reflect the efforts by patients literally to survive.

Undertreated or otherwise uncontrolled pain can worsen aberrant behavior. All patients treated for chronic pain are at risk for aberrant behavior, regardless of whether they are also at risk for addiction. This is because chronic pain engenders great stress, disengagement from society, estrangement from family and friends, and financial trouble. Most patients living with moderate-to-severe pain find that performing the simple chores of daily life is an unending challenge. Pain relief is elusive and seems unattainable. Chronic pain also creates changes in the central nervous system that are similar to those caused by anxiety and depression. Over time, these circumstances lead to despair.

Chemical Coping

At a congressional hearing on crime, Representative Shirley Chisholm spoke of substance abuse as "the need to escape from harsh reality."[15] A patient who copes chemically with life's challenges is unwisely seeking escape from his or her own overwhelming psychologic stress. Anxiety, depression, posttraumatic stress disorder, or another mental disease such as bipolar disorder or schizophrenia can trigger chemical coping. For example, a person with borderline personality disorder may self-medicate to moderate feelings of fear, anger, or boredom. An insomniac might overuse opioids in an attempt to sleep. Pain can be a stressor, as can financial worries or a weak social support system. Medications other than opioids may also be abused, sometimes in combination. Chemical copers are especially prone to dangerous drug interactions through the combining of substances. Benzodiazepines and alcohol are frequently identified in combination in overdose deaths.

Chemical coping is invariably a resounding failure. The patient's function and quality of life continue to sink deeper into unmanageable territory as the chemical abuse worsens. A certain impulsive quality to drug use is characteristic. The coper's symptoms of mental disease may worsen in the absence of the proper diagnosis and treatment. Such persons often display strong emotional reactions and a marked inability to handle life's challenges.

For some chemical copers, pain has become secondary. A few may exhibit somatoform disorder or physical symptoms rooted in psychologic rather than physical causes. Unfortunately, healthcare systems sometimes provide little financial support for psychiatric and behavioral therapies and inadvertently encourage these patients to "stay sick" within the traditional medical system.

For many more chemical copers, pain is a persistent factor that is worsened by anxiety, depression, or another mental disease. The painful symptoms are not "all in the patient's head" but are genuine physiologic byproducts of complicating mental factors.

Opioids are valuable assets in treating pain but are far less effective if they exacerbate a patient's mental troubles. For those patients, pain treatments must be administered in tandem with appropriate psychiatric interventions and medications, behavioral therapies, and education in coping skills, when needed. Clinicians should not hesitate to refer their patients to professionals in these fields.

Rational Abuse

Some patients actually do experience improvement from the misuse of their medications, at least in the short term. This observable occurrence could be called "rational abuse:" medication misuse that improves the patient's function and quality of life. The patient's motive is to successfully control pain, psychiatric symptoms, or other facets of life that he or she believes are mitigated by taking the medication. Such abuse is appropriately termed "rational."

Rational abuse reflects a patient's attempt to feel normal. Most patients of this type who find some degree of physical or psychologic relief by escalating their own doses tend to have mild-to-moderate pain rather than more severe pain. Just because rational abuse is understandable, however, does not mean that it is acceptable. Defying medical direction is dangerous. Such actions must be addressed by the patient's clinician. For example, methadone is sometimes prescribed as an analgesic for chronic pain and must be taken precisely as directed. Methadone stays in the system longer than do most opioids, and patients vary greatly in their metabolic response to it. If patients take an extra dose of methadone (as they may have done with another opioid in the past) they are at risk for death from respiratory depression, particularly if they ingest methadone and another substance that is a central nervous system depressant. Any controlled substance can be hazardous when used outside of medical direction. The answer is for clinicians to monitor patients for compliance with prescribed doses; to make referrals, dose adjustments, or medication changes when needed; and to conduct ongoing assessments of pain relief, function, and quality of life. These measures should eliminate the need for patients to "play doctor" and adjust the doses of their own medication.

Trio Diagnosis: Three Conditions in One

A person who exhibits both a substance-use disorder and a mental disease is said to have a "dual diagnosis." When a chronic-pain condition is added to a dual diagnosis, a new condition is created that could be called a "trio diagnosis" (Figure III:3). It has already been stated that finding a perfect solution for patients with chronic pain can be elusive. When

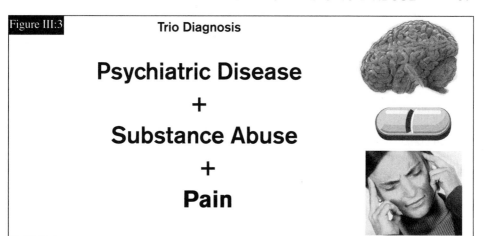

Figure III:3   Trio Diagnosis

Psychiatric Disease
+
Substance Abuse
+
Pain

those individuals also demonstrate a high risk for substance abuse, they are doubly complex. Add the presence of a mental disease, and the result is a daunting interplay of physiologic, neurologic, and psychosocial factors, all of which require medical attention. When a trio diagnosis is present, all 3 conditions must be treated simultaneously. The clinician should not treat only pain and hope that the patient's severe anxiety will resolve in the meantime. Similarly, maintaining an exclusive focus on psychiatric symptoms while an active substance-use disorder rages on will result in little progress. Likewise, an individual who abuses substances is unlikely to stop doing so while battling uncontrolled pain. The likelihood of an improved outcome is severely hampered if all 3 conditions are not addressed in a patient with a trio diagnosis.

Addiction

This is the diagnosis most often suspected and also most feared by the treating clinician. The recognition of an underlying addiction in a patient presenting with chronic pain can be one of the most difficult diagnoses in medicine. However, with time, the clinical skills needed to help these patients can be learned. The presence of aberrant behavior, though an important warning sign, does not alone warrant a diagnosis of addictive disease. However, some characteristics are common in people gripped by an active addiction. Addicted patients are likely to:

- Exhibit multiple aberrant behaviors.
- Indulge in at least 1 highly egregious behavior.
- Defy any efforts to limit their aberrant behavior.
- Remain unresponsive to efforts to improve their pain.
- Lose quality of life and physical function.
- Exhibit a persistent craving for opioids to achieve euphoric or other psychogenic effects.
- Use a substance in a larger amount or for longer periods than intended.
- Display an overwhelming focus on opioids.
- Spend considerable time and effort in the compulsive search for opioids.
- Reduce other activities in social, recreational, or occupational realms.

- Continue to use opioids despite harm to health, social relationships, or finances.
- Return to opioid abuse even after having been successfully weaned. This characteristic strongly suggests an addicted person.

A patient with the disease of addiction needs treatment for that disorder in tandem with pain therapy. It is vital that clinicians realize that the undertreatment of pain may lead to the recurrence of drug-seeking behavior in a recovering addicted patient. Adequate pain control is important to the addicted person's return to healthful functioning. If addiction or a trio diagnosis is suspected, it is good medical practice to obtain more than 1 medical opinion. It is also imperative to refer the patient to experts in addiction medicine and psychiatric specialties as needed. These patients are complex. Trying to effect a cure without help could harm the patient (and ultimately, the clinician's practice).

The Sociology of Abuse

Socioeconomic issues influence the development of aberrant behavior and are often overlooked by practitioners. Consider research in rural Kentucky, where controlled-release oxycodone abuse made headlines in the early 2000s.[16] Many people there have family and societal histories of coal mining, with its attendant problems of painful illnesses and poverty. The moonshine that helped to medicate these ills in the past has been replaced today by pharmaceuticals. It should not go unnoticed that the cost of pain medication is sometimes covered by insurance, so for someone who is struggling with finances, prescribed medication is a more wallet-friendly choice than the purchase of street drugs.

Understanding the Behavior of Abuse

Turning again to the model depicted in Figure III:2, the rationale of patients who engage in egregious behaviors may be the easiest to interpret. The high number and severity of aberrant behaviors identified in patients at the far right of the spectrum are likely to indicate a severe problem with opioid abuse or addiction. Conversely, patients at the far left of the Figure who exhibit no problems with opioid intake, barring 1 or 2 minor aberrant behaviors, are probably obtaining the pain control they seek.

The patients who prove most difficult to manage are those who occupy the middle of the spectrum of Figure III:2. When those patients take more medication than the dose prescribed or in other ways fail to follow the opioid-treatment agreement, their reasons for doing so may be unclear. Indeed, their behavior may be subject to multiple and complex influences. Are they rational abusers, whose conditions will improve as a result of noncompliance? Are they chemically coping with a poor social support system? Is a comorbid disorder such as anxiety or depression to blame? Distinctions may be difficult because the chaos (social, family, and financial) wrought by substance abuse closely resembles the turmoil experienced by some people who live with chronic pain.

Is Your Patient Addicted to Drugs or Abusing Them?

The same genetic, psychosocial, and neurochemical factors that foster addiction also apply to drug abuse, which is far easier to manage via skillful intervention. Clinically distinguishing addiction from drug abuse is not always easy. As stated in the following guidelines published as a consensus of several pain and addiction societies:

It should be emphasized that no single event is diagnostic of addictive disorder. Rather, the diagnosis is made in response to a pattern of behaviors that usually becomes obvious over time.[4]

Many people who are considered to be addicts are really pain patients for whom opioids are ineffective and who desire to cease opioid therapy but cannot face the actual or anticipated pain of physical withdrawal. The result is that such patients "cannot stop" taking the medication. They may believe that they are addicted to their prescribed drugs. Their family and even their treating clinicians may believe that as well. These patients can usually be managed with an alternative pain-control method and the gradual, careful cessation of opioid therapy (see Chapter VI for an exit strategy). If, over time, the clinician realizes that the primary problem is one of substance abuse and not other clinical difficulties stemming from tolerance, uncontrolled pain, or fear of either anticipated pain or the withdrawal of therapy, the abuse is likely to fit one of the categories delineated as follows by Zacny and colleagues:

• Those who abuse only prescription opioids.
• Heroin abusers who abuse opioids when they cannot obtain heroin or another opiate.
• Polydrug abusers who use opioids for an occasional high or to boost the effect of their drug of choice.
• Pain patients who abuse or become dependent on opioids during the course of pain treatment. These patients obtain no medical benefit from their drug use and are not just physically dependent on the drug.[17]

The exact number of patients in this last group is unknown. Few prospective studies have compared the rate of drug abuse in chronic-pain patients with that in other patients, with or without a history of substance abuse. What is known, however, is that pain may interact with substance abuse in complex ways. A higher prevalence of chronic pain has been observed among persons being treated for substance-use disorders.[18] A small but significant percent of chronic-pain sufferers have at one time or another turned to alcohol for pain relief.[19] It is important to examine the underlying motivations that drive such syndromes, because the patient may need treatment for comorbid disorders. When assessing patients, clinicians should be cognizant of and guard against overidentifying their own "pet" diagnosis, whether that is uncontrolled pain, addictive disease, or something else.

Screening for Aberrant Behavior

Many aberrant drug-related behaviors go unnoticed by clinicians and can be difficult to verify, even when suspected. A report of aberrant behavior is usually noted in 1 of 3 ways:

• It is observed by clinicians or office staff during clinical interaction with the patient.
• It is obtained from objective sources, such as a prescription-monitoring database, the results of drug screening, or a law-enforcement report.
• It is obtained via verbal reports by the patient, the patient's family and friends, pharmacists, or other interested parties.

To be useful indicators of a patient's compliance with opioid therapy, measurements of aberrant drug-related behavior should be:

- *Verified as accurate to the extent possible.* This might involve requesting files from previous providers, performing drug screenings of the patient's blood or urine, and/or querying state prescription-monitoring databases.
- *Monitored over time.* Physicians must screen for and document aberrant drug-related behaviors during every clinic visit.
- *Addressed as they are noted.* For every aberrant behavior displayed, a clinical solution should be presented to the patient. The consequences of noncompliance must be clearly outlined (see information on opioid treatment agreements in Chapter VI).
- *Monitored for improvement.* If no improvement is observed after a reasonable attempt to manage the aberrant behavior, it is time to discuss alternative therapies, to refer the patient to treatment for addiction, to outline psychiatric interventions, or to introduce other suitable measures that may ultimately include discharge from the clinician's care.

Subjective Versus Objective Reports

Some aberrant behaviors that are more evidence-based than others can be identified by established signs (eg, cocaine in the patient's urine, opioids prescribed by multiple providers for the same person, frequent visits to a hospital emergency department to obtain opioids) that can be verified objectively (by drug screening, a report from a prescription-monitoring system, or a check of medical records, respectively). Many aberrant behaviors (visible intoxication, requesting early refills, resisting therapy) can be observed in the clinical setting. Some behaviors (reports of stealing or borrowing medications from others, buying drugs from street sources, the concurrent abuse of alcohol) are revealed during conversations with the patient or his or her family and friends. These categories may overlap; for example, drug procurement from street sources may be reported subjectively or may be verified objectively through drug screening.

Although objective verifiable reports of drug abuse are preferred by most clinicians, a subjective verbal report can also provide valuable information. The patient may not volunteer that he or she is using street drugs but is the best source for a description of lifestyle chaos and stress. Family members may be the first to identify a problem with medication overuse in their loved one, and their concerns are well worth listening to. If the family system is dysfunctional in some manner (for example, if the patient's family members believe that all consumption of opioids leads to addiction or if a family environment of substance abuse leads members to want to share the patient's prescriptions), these patterns are often revealed in conversation. This type of monitoring takes a willingness to listen with care and insight.

Patient Management: There Is No Risk-Free Treatment

There is always a possibility that by prescribing opioids, a clinician may unwittingly contribute to a patient's serious drug abuse problem. Because opioids are potentially addictive substances, they carry a risk that must be managed if patients are to receive the pain relief they deserve. No medical therapy is risk free, and pain treatments other than opioids contribute their own potential dangers. For example, the use of nonsteroidal anti-inflammatory drugs is linked to an estimated 16,500 deaths every year in the United States among patients with rheumatoid arthritis or osteoarthritis.[20]

Tools, Not Labels

We have been examining various categories of motivation for drug abuse. While useful, those categories are not intended to be used as strict interpretations of individual behavior. It is human nature to try to categorize any challenge to better understand and conquer it. However, labels applied to humans have a way of "coming unstuck." The behavior of patients may blend characteristics from several such categories, or it may change categories as life circumstances change. It is crucial not to label a person who abuses chemical substances as "addicted" for lack of a better understanding of his or her condition. Conversely, failure to treat addiction when it is present can encourage a person to continue destructive and potentially deadly behavior.

The information on patient behavior in Box III:5 can help clinicians to take appropriate action if drug abuse is suspected. A compliant patient whose pain is well treated with opioids exhibits increased function and an improved quality of life but exhibits little or no aberrant behavior. The addicted patient engages in multiple or egregious behaviors and experiences a diminished quality of life and function after inappropriate drug use. The behavior of patients who fit in the moderate-behavior category can usually be managed, but those individuals are the most difficult to assess. Inappropriate drug use may be the result of an attempt to cope or to manage uncontrolled pain, or it may reflect rational abuse, and the patient's function and quality of life may either improve or decline after inappropriate medication use. The example in Box III:6 is an exercise in patient assessment. What if this patient presented for treatment in your office? The questions raised provide a good place to start in the evaluation of any patient.

Box III:5	Spectrum of Patient Behaviors with Long-Term Opioid Therapy		
Compliant Patient	**Chemical Coper? Rational Abuser? Uncontrolled Pain Patient?**	**Addicted Patient**	
No or few aberrant behaviors	Moderate aberrant behavior	Egregious behavior or multiple aberrant behaviors	
Appropriate use	Inappropriate use	Inappropriate use	
Quality of life ⬆	Quality of life ⬆ or ⬇	Quality of life ⬇	
Function ⬆	Function ⬆ or ⬇	Function ⬇	

Box III:6   ## Suppose this patient came for treatment?

How should he be managed?

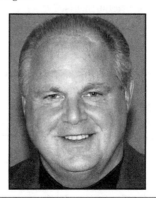

Name: LIMBAUGH, RUSH HUDSON	**Race:** White
Address:	**DOB:** 01/12/1951
	Facility: MDC INTAKE
OBTS Number: N/A	**Booking Number:** 2006021379
Arresting Agency: 01 - PBSO	**Booking Date:** 04/28/2006 Time: 16:25
Original Bond: $3,000.00	**Officer:** J. HOFFMAN
Release Date: N/A	**Current Bond:** $3,000.00
Warrant Number: N/A	**Holds For Other Agencies:** No

Charges:
893.13-3730   FRAUD-CONCEAL INFO TO OBTAIN PRESCRIPTION

What Is Known (or Has Been Published) About This Patient

- He suffered pain after unsuccessful back surgery.
- He abused large quantities of prescription opioids for several years.
- He kept the abuse secret from wife, colleagues, and friends.
- He twice entered a rehabilitation program, but his abuse recurred.
- While abusing drugs, he remained successful without a visible reduction in functioning.
- He is suspected of buying pills illegally.

What Is Not Known About This Patient

- Whether he has a history of substance abuse.
- Whether he has an undiagnosed psychiatric disorder.
- His main motivation for drug-seeking behavior. Is it:

    - To control physical pain?
    - To mask emotional pain or stress?
    - To seek a "high?"
    - Some combination of those reasons?

Law-enforcement and other regulatory agencies sometimes take an overriding interest in determining whether patients are addicted. Clinicians, realizing that a good clinical outcome is unlikely in the presence of an active addiction, should focus on the goals of ensuring improved pain relief, physical function, and quality of life. When the patient is monitored with these goals in mind and with a commitment to diagnosing any complicating comorbid conditions, pain treatment has a far greater chance of success.

Conclusion

People misuse medications for many reasons, only one of which is an active addictive disorder. People abuse their prescriptions because they want to solve their problems, to relieve pain or feel less anxious, to find oblivion, or to fit in with their social circles. The need to watch for aberrant behavior does not mean that a clinician is legally obligated to always be right about a patient's motivations and can never be fooled. Physicians and other healthcare professionals assess their patients for opioid compliance to ensure the efficacy of pain treatment and to diagnose and treat any possible complicating disorders. They are not responsible for any patient's choice to behave irresponsibly or criminally.

The careful observation and documentation of drug-related aberrant behavior should be charted as are other clinical data, such as the level of hemoglobin A1c in diabetic patients or the blood pressure value in those with hypertension. As detailed in the following chapters, it is even possible to identify the patients who are at highest risk for potential drug abuse problems before opioid therapy is initiated.

References

1. Burglass ME, Shaffer H. Diagnosis in the addictions I: conceptual problems. In: *The Addictive Behaviors*. Shaffer H, Stimmel B, eds. New York, NY: Haworth Press; 1984.
2. Webster LR, Webster RM. Predicting aberrant behaviors in opioid-treated patients: preliminary validation of the Opioid Risk Tool. Pain Med. 2005 Nov-Dec;6(6):432-42.
3. Passik SD, Kirsh KL, Whitcomb L, Portenoy RK, Katz NP, Kleinman L, Dodd SL, Schein JR. A new tool to assess and document pain outcomes in chronic pain patients receiving opioid therapy. Clin Ther. 2004 Apr;26(4):552-61.
4. American Academy of Pain Medicine, American Pain Society, and American Society of Addiction Medicine. Definitions related to the use of opioids for the treatment of pain: consensus document. Under review. Glenview, IL and Chevy Chase, MD; 2001.
5. Passik SD, Kirsh KL, Whitcomb L, Dickerson PK, Theobald DE. Pain clinicians' rankings of aberrant drug-taking behaviors. J Pain Palliat Care Pharmacother. 2002;16(4):39-49.
6. Compton P, Darakjian J, Miotto K. Screening for addiction in patients with chronic pain and "problematic" substance use: evaluation of a pilot assessment tool. J Pain Symptom Manage. 1998 Dec;16(6):355-63.
7. Chabal C, Erjavec MK, Jacobson L, Mariano A, Chaney E. Prescription opiate abuse in chronic pain patients: clinical criteria, incidence, and predictors. Clin J Pain. 1997 Jun;13(2):150-5.

8. Passik SD, Kirsh KL, Whitcomb L, Schein JR, Kaplan MA, Dodd SL, Kleinman L, Katz NP, Portenoy RK. Monitoring outcomes during long-term opioid therapy for noncancer pain: results with the Pain Assessment and Documentation Tool. J Opioid Manag. 2005 Nov-Dec;1(5):257-66.

9. Berndt S, Maier C, Schutz HW. Polymedication and medication compliance in patients with chronic non-malignant pain. Pain. 1993 Mar;52(3):331-9.

10. Kell M. Monitoring compliance with OxyContin prescriptions in 14,712 patients treated in 127 outpatient pain centers. Pain Med. 2005; 6(2):186-7.

11. Reid MC, Engles-Horton LL, Weber MB, Kerns RD, Rogers EL, O'Connor PG. Use of opioid medications for chronic noncancer pain syndromes in primary care. J Gen Intern Med. 2002 Mar;17(3):173-9.

12. Robinson RC, Gatchel RJ, Polatin P, Deschner M, Noe C, Gajraj N. Screening for problematic prescription opioid use. Clin J Pain. 2001 Sep;17(3):220-8.

13. Kirsh KL, Whitcomb LA, Donaghy K, Passik SD. Abuse and addiction issues in medically ill patients with pain: attempts at clarification of terms and empirical study. Clin J Pain 2002 Jul-Aug;18(14 Suppl):S52-60.

14. Weissman DE, Haddox JD. Opioid pseudoaddiction—an iatrogenic syndrome. Pain. 1989 Mar;36(3):363-6.

15. Quotes by Shirley Chisholm. Answers.com Web site. Available at: http://www.answers.com/topic/shirley-chisholm. Accessed April 10, 2007.

16. Hays LR. A profile of OxyContin addiction. J Addict Dis 2004; 23(4):1-9.

17. Zacny J, Bigelow G, Compton P, Foley K, Iguchi M, Sannerud C. College on Problems of Drug Dependence taskforce on prescription opioid non-medical use and abuse: position statement. Drug Alcohol Depend. 2003 Apr 1;69(3):215-32.

18. Rosenblum A, Joseph H, Fong C, Kipnis S, Cleland C, Portenoy RK. Prevalence and characteristics of chronic pain among chemically dependent patients in methadone maintenance and residential treatment facilities. JAMA. 2003 May 14;289(18):2370-8.

19. Chronic Pain In America: Roadblocks To Relief. Research conducted for the American Pain Society, the American Academy of Pain Medicine and Janssen Pharmaceutica by Roper Starch Worldwide Inc., January 1999. American Pain Society Web site. Available http://www.ampainsoc.org/whatsnew/conclude_road.htm. Accessed March 2, 2004.

20. Wolfe MM, Lichtenstein DR, Singh G. Gastrointestinal toxicity of nonsteroidal anti-inflammatory drugs. N Engl J Med. 1999;340(24):1888–99.

CHAPTER IV

RISK FACTORS FOR OPIOID ABUSE

It is much more important to know what sort of a patient has a disease than what sort of a disease a patient has.
-William Osler, MD, former professor and physician-in-chief, Johns Hopkins Hospital[1]

A certain number of people in pain will eventually exhibit symptoms of drug abuse or addiction. However, not every patient is at equal risk for abuse or addiction. This chapter will examine the risk factors for drug abuse with the goal of understanding the reasons why some patients are more vulnerable than others. Because abusers of 1 category of substance are at risk for abusing substances in other categories, the misuse of alcohol, illegal drugs, and prescription opioids is examined. The risk profile of an abuser frequently includes complications such as mental disease or polysubstance abuse. The ways in which those factors are interrelated and mutually reinforcing are considered.

Individual Risk Factors for Substance Abuse

According to a popular misconception, all patients are equally likely to abuse opioids prescribed for the treatment of chronic pain. Opioid prescribing is presumed to be a gamble during which patients might win a better life or lose their well-being to the disease of addiction at a toss of the dice. Scientific evidence refutes that concept, however. In fact, certain risk factors for an increased risk of opioid abuse in patients have been well documented. Knowing in advance whether a patient possesses these risk factors can assist a clinician in monitoring the progress of treatment. Some of the risk factors for opioid abuse, which have been gleaned from the scientific literature and clinical practice, include:

• A personal history of substance abuse.[2]
• A family history of substance abuse.[2]
• Young age.[2]
• A history of preadolescent sexual abuse.[2]
• Mental disease.[2]
• Social patterns of drug use.[3]
• Psychologic stress.[3]
• Failure to participate in a 12-step program.[4]
• Polysubstance abuse.[4]
• Poor social support.[4]
• Cigarette dependency.[5]
• A history of repeated drug and/or alcohol rehabilitation.[5]
• A focus on opioids.[6]
• Nonfunctional status caused by pain.[6]
• Exaggeration of pain.[6]
• Unclear cause of pain.[6]

Among clinicians and researchers, no consensus exists regarding the risk factors that are most predictive of drug abuse. Such evidence is far from conclusive, even for the best-documented risk factors, and the quality of research varies. For example, in 1 study, past opiate abuse and depressive symptoms failed to predict which subjects would abuse opioids.[7] This should serve to remind us that whatever a patient's history or level of risk, we can only estimate whether a patient is likely to abuse opioids; we cannot know for certain that he or she will do so. However, the characteristics listed below have been identified as strongly supported predictors of drug abuse:

A personal history of substance abuse (alcohol, illegal drugs, or prescription drugs)

This is perhaps the most important risk factor for substance abuse. Clinical observation and published studies have shown that patients with a history of abusing prescriptions or illegal drugs are likely to continue their substance abuse and aberrant behavior. The risk for future problems with opioid intake is greatest when the history of abuse is recent and involves multiple substances. The risk becomes more significant still when the history of abuse involves prescription opioids or other opiates. In a study of shared vulnerability for

Box IV:1	**Shared Vulnerability of Different Categories of Drugs**				
	Probability of Drug Abuse (N = 6744)				
Index Drug	**Marijuana**	**Stimulants**	**Sedatives**	**Heroin & Opiates**	**Psyche-delics**
Marijuana	NA	.31	.12	.07	.12
Stimulants	.52	NA	.17	.11	.18
Sedatives	.63	.53	NA	.20	.26
Heroin and opiates	.46	.44	.26	NA	.14
Psychedelic agents	.80	.72	.32	.14	NA

NA = Not applicable.

Source: Tsuang MT, Lyons MJ, Meyer JM, Doyle T, Eisen SA, Goldberg J, True W, Lin N, Toomey R, Eaves L. Co-occurrence of abuse of different drugs in men: the role of drug-specific and shared vulnerabilities. Arch Gen Psychiatry. 1998 Nov;55(11):967-72.

drug abuse, abusers of 1 category of drugs exhibited a high degree of abuse of different categories (Box IV:1).[8] That risk was relative. For example, opioid abuse was poorly correlated with marijuana intake but had slightly more correlation with the abuse of stimulants. Each drug studied (with the exception of psychedelic agents) demonstrated its own unique genetic influences specific to the use of that drug only (Box IV:2). Heroin (and presumably other opiates) shared fewer genetic influences with other drugs than did any other agent studied, which suggests that most of the genetic influence in opiate abuse is specific to opiates. Conversely, individuals who abused marijuana, stimulants, sedatives, or psychedelic drugs exhibited no greater than a 20% probability of experiencing an opioid-related substance-abuse problem. That evidence relegates prior opiate abuse to a category of its own and marks it as a strong predictor of future opiate abuse.

Though less significant than opiate abuse, the prior abuse of nonopioid illegal drugs or alcohol also increases the risk for problems with the abuse of prescription opioids. Individuals who abuse 1 substance are 7 times more likely than others to abuse an additional substance.[9] One study of personal polysubstance abuse showed that most individuals who were admitted to a healthcare facility for alcohol treatment had also abused 1 or more additional substances in the 3 months before their admission for alcohol treatment.[10]

The personal-history warning signs for potential opioid abuse can be arranged in the following hierarchy from most to least dangerous:

Box IV:2   Genetic Influences on Specific Drugs of Abuse

Variance in Drug Abuse Variables from Multivariate Biometrical Modeling (Latent Phenotype Model)

Substance Categories	Total Genetic Variance
Marijuana	0.33
Stimulants	0.33
Sedatives	0.27
Heroin and opiates	0.54
Psychedelic agents	0.26

Source: Tsuang MT, Lyons MJ, Meyer JM, Doyle T, Eisen SA, Goldberg J, True W, Lin N, Toomey R, Eaves L. Co-occurrence of abuse of different drugs in men: the role of drug-specific and shared vulnerabilities. Arch Gen Psychiatry. 1998 Nov;55(11):967-72.

- Prescription opioid and/or opiate abuse (including heroin).
- Polysubstance abuse.
- Abuse of other illegal drugs.
- Extreme abuse of alcohol.

It may appear that the "illegal drug" category is compromised by the presence of marijuana, which has a low correlation to opioid abuse, but it is reasonable to posit that marijuana, as an illegal drug, is likely to be consumed in a household more tolerant of polysubstance abuse than in a household in which marijuana is not used. Such careful delineations should not obscure the fact that any past or current substance abuse is a risk factor for problems with the future abuse of prescription opioids.

Family history of substance abuse (alcohol, illegal drugs or prescription drugs)
A family history of substance abuse can confer both genetic and environmental risks for the development of substance abuse.[11] The attitudes of parents or other family role models toward the use or misuse of illicit and prescription drugs can establish a permissive environment in which substance abuse is tolerated or encouraged. As noted previously, opiate abuse appears strongly dependent on a genetic influence. Thus a patient's family history of any kind of opiate abuse may be a strong risk factor for his or her abuse of prescribed opioids.[12]

The frequent crossover from 1 drug of abuse to another is reason to consider the abuse of substances other than opioids as risk factors for future opioid abuse. For example, a tendency to become addicted to alcohol is considered a "family disease" because it occurs in generations of the same family. Alcoholism is 2 to 4 times more likely to occur in the close relative of a treated alcoholic than in the close relative of a nonalcoholic.[13] One could say that alcoholism is not a strong risk factor for opioid abuse, because a relatively weak correlation exists between a family history of alcoholism and later opioid abuse in an individual. However, a family problem with alcoholism can create a dynamic in which polysubstance abuse occurs and may foster an environment in which opioid abuse is a possible outcome.

Young Age
In general, youth is a risk factor for substance abuse. The onset of drug abuse often occurs at a very early age. From middle-to-late adolescence into the mid-20s appears to be the time at which most drug experimentation occurs. In a survey by the National Institute of Mental Health (NIMH) of 4778 respondents, 22.3% of people age 18 to 30 years had a substance-use disorder.[14] US statistics show that the abuse of drugs other than alcohol declines as people age.[15] Furthermore, many mental disorders, which are strongly linked to substance abuse, are first manifested in youth (Figure IV:1). The onset of major depression usually occurs during the decade from midadolescence to the mid-20s. According to the results of the NIMH survey, a major depressive episode or anxiety disorder was associated with double the risk of a subsequent drug disorder in young people age 18 to 30 years.[14] Of those with multiple mental disorders, 80% reported the onset of a substance-use disorder before the age of 20 years.

With respect to opioids administered for pain, age confers another liability as well. Recent data suggest that a tolerance to opioids develops much more quickly in younger indi-

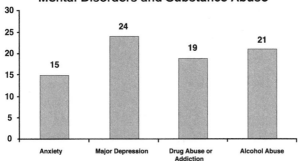

Psychologic Disease: Median Age for Onset of Mental Disorders and Substance Abuse

Source: Christie KA, Burke JD Jr, Regier DA, Rae DS, Boyd JH, Locke BZ. Epidemiologic evidence for early onset of mental disorders and higher risk of drug abuse in young adults. Am J Psychiatry. 1988 Aug;145(8):971-5.

viduals.[16] Researchers at the University of California at San Francisco found that in patients younger than 50 years who had nerve damage, achieving pain relief from arthritis or fibromyalgia required more than twice the morphine-equivalent dose as that needed by patients older than 60 years. The younger patients also reported less long-term pain relief. The researchers theorized that age-related changes in neurons could be to blame for causing younger patients to achieve physical tolerance more rapidly and therefore to need more medication to achieve relief. If that theory is supported by subsequent research, young people may be at risk for aberrant "drug-seeking" behaviors that resemble drug abuse or addictive disease but are instead the pursuit of pain relief.

Although age is 1 risk factor for medication misuse, its importance can be assessed only as part of a cumulative risk-factor profile. In the presence of other risk factors (eg, preadolescent sexual abuse, a mental disorder, intense stressors, a social environment that fosters medication misuse), age becomes a predictor for drug abuse. However, it should not be assumed that every youthful patient is likely to exhibit abuse, nor should it be assumed that older patients will not.

History of Preadolescent Sexual Abuse

A history of sexual mistreatment is common in people who abuse substances.[17] Much of that trauma occurs during childhood. Research involving women who seek substance-abuse treatment and who also have a history of physical or sexual trauma indicates that most had been abused by the age of 18 years.

A 10-year study of female twins showed that depression, anxiety, panic disorders, and alcohol and drug dependency all increased following preadolescent sexual abuse (Figure IV:2).[18] Of all the disorders measured, drug dependency occurred most frequently after sexual abuse. In another study of 286 women, about 9% of the subjects studied reported having been victims of childhood sexual abuse, and of that group, 64% had been treated for depression during a 3-year period.[19] The authors of that study concluded that a history

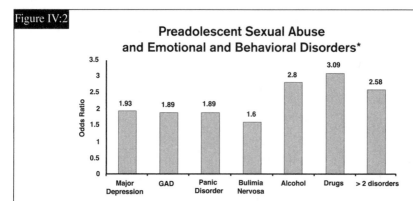

Figure IV:2

Preadolescent Sexual Abuse and Emotional and Behavioral Disorders*

N = 1411 Adult female twins
GAD - Generalized Anxiety Disorder
Source: Kendler KS, Bulik CM, Silberg J, Hettema JM, Myers J, Prescott CA. Childhood sexual abuse and adult psychiatric and substance use disorders in women: an epidemiological and cotwin control analysis. Arch Gen Psychiatry. 2000 Oct;57(10):953-9.

of sexual abuse is probably a contributing factor to depression. The depression and anxiety that develop after sexual abuse are strong risk factors for subsequent substance abuse.

Another condition that develops after preadolescent sexual abuse is posttraumatic stress disorder (PTSD). PTSD is severe anxiety resulting from a prior event that caused extreme terror and feelings of helplessness and involved death, serious injury, or physical threat to the self or others. It is a frequent comorbid diagnosis with drug abuse. Women exhibit that comorbid diagnosis more often than do men: of women in drug-abuse treatment, 30% to 59% also have PTSD.[20] This rate is 2 to 3 times that in men seeking drug-abuse treatment.

Boys also experience preadolescent abuse, though at a frequency far less than that of girls, and girls are more likely to develop PTSD after molestation than are boys.[20] In all people who are sexually abused, the emotional damage can be persistent and severe. The rate of PTSD is actually higher in men who have been raped than in women who have been raped; however, women are 10 times more likely to be raped than are men.[21]

The experience of preadolescent sexual abuse is uniquely traumatic and is distinctively associated with substance abuse later in life. Trauma-induced anxiety, whether conscious or unconscious, is a powerful stimulus to seek relief from disturbing memories. The anxiolysis sought from drugs and alcohol is an unfortunate common result.

Mental Disease

The contribution of mental disease to substance abuse should not be underestimated, particularly in the United States, which leads the world in reported mental disorders. The NIMH reports that 25% of the US population experiences symptoms that suggest the diagnosis of a mental disorder and that almost 50% of all Americans will experience some form of mental illness during their lifetime.[22-23] The link between mental disease and substance abuse is well established. The NIMH interviewed more than 20,000 individuals and found that of those with a lifelong diagnosis of a mental disorder, 22.3% exhibited alcohol abuse or addiction and 14.7% exhibited drug abuse or addiction.[9] Among those with no history of a mental disorder, the rate of alcohol abuse was 11% and the rate of drug abuse was 3.7%. Thus having a lifelong mental disorder is associated with twice the risk of having an alcohol disorder and with 4 times the risk of having another drug-abuse disorder. The individuals studied were interviewed in a community setting and were not part of a treatment-seeking population who, it is supposed, would report even higher rates of concomitant disorders. Psychiatric illnesses are common in patients who are undergoing treatment for drug abuse, and that type of illness should be considered in the management of those individuals. Approximately 6 of 10 patients being treated for substance abuse also exhibit mental illness, and 25% to 60% of individuals with a mental illness also abuse substances, according to NIDA.[24]

The link between mental disease and substance abuse is found in other countries as well. The United Kingdom reports an incidence of psychiatric disorders among drug-dependent subjects that is 3 times higher than that among subjects who are not drug dependent.[25] This was true even after controlling for such social and demographic factors as age, ethnicity, housing status, and employment status.

Substance Abuse and Specific Mental Disorders

Evidence from the NIMH that links specific mental disorders to substance abuse is striking (Figure IV:3).[9] Almost 25% of the subjects with an anxiety disorder had a concomitant substance-use disorder. When phobias, which have a high prevalence in the US general population, were not considered, one sees even more co-occurrence with substance abuse: 35.8% of subjects with panic disorder and 32.8% of subjects with obsessive-compulsive disorder had a substance-use disorder. An individual with schizophrenia was 4.6 times more likely to have a substance-use disorder than was someone without schizophrenia. Substance abuse was identified in 83.6% of people with antisocial personality disorder,

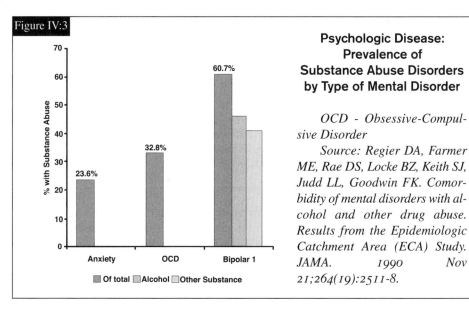

Figure IV:3

Psychologic Disease: Prevalence of Substance Abuse Disorders by Type of Mental Disorder

OCD - Obsessive-Compulsive Disorder

Source: Regier DA, Farmer ME, Rae DS, Locke BZ, Keith SJ, Judd LL, Goodwin FK. Comorbidity of mental disorders with alcohol and other drug abuse. Results from the Epidemiologic Catchment Area (ECA) Study. JAMA. 1990 Nov 21;264(19):2511-8.

which lists substance abuse as a major criterion for its diagnosis. Bipolar I disorder was associated with an extraordinary risk of substance abuse (11 times greater than that in people without the disorder). Alcohol and drug dependence were more than twice as common in bipolar patients than in patients with unipolar depression. However, patients with unipolar depression were at greater risk for substance abuse than were members of the general US population. Depression is also a likely factor in relapse to drug abuse.

A diagnosis of attention-deficit hyperactivity disorder (ADHD) in childhood can also confer an amplified risk of alcohol and substance abuse later in life. For 4 years, Boston researchers followed 212 boys, some of whom had ADHD.[26] Of those with ADHD, some were receiving medication and others were not treated. The researchers discovered that 75% of the boys who received no medication for their ADHD began using marijuana, alcohol, hallucinogens, stimulants, or cocaine during the 4-year study period. Only 25% of the medicated boys and 18% of the boys without ADHD abused those substances. ADHD also increases the likelihood of anxiety and mood disorders that can exacerbate problematic drug use.

Sex Differences in Drug Abusers with Mental Disease

The mental diseases that occur concomitantly with substance abuse are not evenly distributed between men and women. Evidence suggests that men are more likely to exhibit antisocial personality disorder than are women, but women are more likely to experience depression or PTSD caused by childhood abuse.[13] This holds true for abusers of alcohol and other drugs. Women are more likely than men to display a comorbid mental diagnosis, though men who abuse substances are far more likely to exhibit a mental disorder than are men in the general population.[27]

Further research could form the basis of gender-specific modalities for the treatment of drug abuse. The role of sexual trauma in women and the greater tendency of men to act on dangerous impulses are just 2 of the dynamics that highlight the need for such a therapeutic approach.

Mental Disease: The Cause or Effect of Substance Abuse?

The strong correlation of mental disease with uncontrolled substance use renders the diagnosis of a mental disorder a risk factor for opioid abuse. Whether mental disease causes substance-use disorders or is caused by them is not clear-cut. For example, some patients become depressed because of the physical and psychologic suffering associated with drug abuse. Others abuse substances to ease the pain of preexisting depression or other mood disorders. Still others experience drug abuse and depression simultaneously. These closely intertwined disorders may originate from common genetic vulnerabilities and may influence each other in a circular behavioral pattern. Again, sex differences may apply. In women, psychiatric factors often seem to precede substance abuse. In men, some evidence suggests that substance abuse often predates the diagnosis of depression, at least in cocaine abusers.[28] It is even possible that a common genetic liability is more likely to be manifested as depression in women and as substance abuse in men because of sex-specific social mores.[13] Far more research is needed to better understand the factors that influence the propensity of a person with a mental illness to abuse substances.

First and foremost, the challenge is to recognize and diagnose drug abuse and mental disorders in patients, some of whom may be seeking medical care for seemingly unrelated physical symptoms. This responsibility often falls to the frontline clinician, who may be the patient's first or only professional medical contact. After diagnosing a substance-use disorder, a mental disorder or both, networking with specialists in addiction and mental health is a must. The results of research are clear: The early recognition and treatment of mental disease are vital to the prevention of prescription opioid abuse.

Is Pain a Risk Factor for Substance Abuse?

One suspected risk factor for opioid abuse — pain itself — is quite controversial. Patient advocates and pain specialists often explain drug abuse by pain patients as the attempt to self-medicate to relieve uncontrolled pain. Thus pain is believed to predate substance abuse, and quite often this is so. However, pain is very prevalent in addicted populations. Just as substance-abuse patients are more likely than others to show symptoms of mental disease, they also report more physical ailments and pain. Research has found approximately twice the rate of lower back pain, headache, and arthritis in substance-abuse patients than in others.[29] The prevalence of pain is particularly high among established abusers of opiates. In a study of patients receiving methadone for chemical dependency, 37% experienced chronic severe pain.[30] Were those individuals self-medicating for pain before their drug abuse or addiction developed? Did the opioid consumed to treat pain trigger a silent drug abuse problem? Were they lying about their pain symptoms to obtain narcotics, or is it possible that chronic pain, which affects the central nervous system, is indeed a risk factor for the development of abuse problems? Perhaps the mechanisms that render a person vulnerable to developing substance abuse also increase the propensity to experience uncontrolled pain.

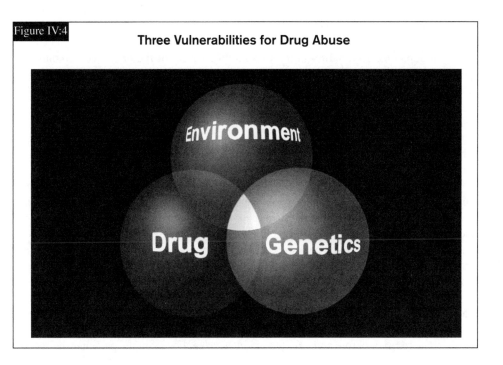

Figure IV:4

Three Vulnerabilities for Drug Abuse

Whichever mechanism or mechanisms are involved, many substance abusers experience unresolved pain, and it is important to understand the association. Perhaps the possibility should not be dismissed quickly that chronic pain itself, with the stress and lifestyle changes it brings, could lead to the uncontrolled abuse of opioids to serve no medical purpose in certain vulnerable individuals. The danger is that this concept could be misunderstood and overapplied to justify the undertreatment of pain and the automatic judging of any aggressive attempt to achieve more pain relief as nonmedical drug seeking.

Vulnerabilities to Substance Abuse

The following 3 types of vulnerability contribute to the likelihood of substance abuse (Figure IV:4):

- The drug itself.
- The environment (both in-home and out-of-home).
- Genetics.

Vulnerabilities show how the cards are stacked but do not assure the game will play out as dealt - in other words, a vulnerability is not a certainty. Genetics appears to exert the strongest influence of those 3 vulnerabilities, and environment is the next strongest influence. Clinical observation indicates that drug properties are the least influential of the 3 vulnerabilities listed.

The Drug

Pharmaceutical companies manufacture and market thousands of different drugs each year, but only a few are associated with substance-use disorders. Potentially addictive drugs have very special properties. It is clear that the reinforcing effects of all drugs of abuse result from dopamine stimulation in the mesolimbic system of the brain. The amount and speed at which dopamine is exposed to the reward center of the brain are determined primarily by the pharmacokinetics of the drug and manner of use.

Pharmacokinetics

The term "pharmacokinetics" refers to the way in which a drug is absorbed and distributed in the host body. The pharmacokinetics of opioids influences how much dopamine is released into the mesolimbic dopamine system.

Two factors primarily account for the "size of the reward" experienced by an opioid-naïve individual: the amount of dopamine released and the speed at which it is released. The greater the amount of dopamine and the more rapid the release, the more likely the drug-induced reward. Heroin for example, quickly triggers the release of a substantial amount of dopamine that delivers a quick peak experience. Extreme peaks are typical of drugs that generate cravings and compulsive use. Slower-release compounds do not provide that same "spike."

The potency of an opioid is related to the amount of dopamine released and how directly that dopamine stimulates the mu receptors. Morphine is a pure mu agonist and a potent opioid. The amount of dopamine released is also affected by the difference in opioid concentration at the receptor before and after the opioid is taken. For example, patients who receive sustained-released morphine around the clock require more morphine to produce a high than do opioid-naive patients.

After a drug has entered the bloodstream, lipophilicity affects the speed at which it enters the brain. Heroin is favored by abusers because it is lipophilic and rapidly enters the brain to stimulate the release of dopamine. Buprenorphine is another very lipophilic opioid that produces less of a high because it only partially stimulates the mu receptor. The rate of decline in opioid blood levels (the "valley" that occurs after the peak experience) also appears to be associated with the potential of a specific opioid for abuse. In general, the sharper the decline in the blood levels of a drug, the stronger the motivation in vulnerable individuals to seek another serving as soon as possible.

Manner of Use

The frequency of use and the route of administration are powerful factors that affect whether the consumption of a drug that is likely to be abused will become reinforcing and destructive. Frequent repeated administration of an opioid for the purpose of obtaining a high is termed "binge use." For a binge user, the intervals between drug uses are short. In an addiction-prone person, this pattern of use leads to craving and compulsive use despite harm. Binge use can increase the risk of abuse, even in individuals who are not genetically susceptible to opioid addiction. This fact does not suggest that the frequent use of an opioid to treat breakthrough pain increases the risk of opioid addiction. The use of an opioid for the treatment of breakthrough pain is intended to produce analgesia, not a high.

The route of drug administration determines in part how quickly dopamine is released. The descending order by route of administration from the quickest to slowest speed of onset for most drugs is as follows: intravenous, inhalational, transmucosal, oral, transdermal. Altering a drug formulation may dramatically change the speed of onset. For example, controlled-release oxycodone, when used as directed, has a slow onset of action and produces a blood level that is sustained for 8 to 12 hours. When the drug is crushed and either chewed or snorted in defiance of medical direction, the abuser experiences a more rapid onset of drug action. Intravenous injection and inhaling are the quickest routes to the reward sought by addicts and abusers.

Short-Acting Opioids Versus Long-Acting Opioids

The drug properties of short-acting opioids (SAOs) are frequently suspected of inciting drug abuse. Many authors and lecturers on the subject of abuse prevention advise clinicians to prescribe long-acting opioids (LAOs) whenever possible to reduce the risk. However, "short acting" refers to the duration of action, not the speed of onset, and it is the speed of onset and subsequent drop-off that constitute the greatest pharmacokinetic factor for misuse. SAOs are frequently misunderstood to be rapid-onset drugs. Actually, most SAOs do not reach a peak effect until 20 to 40 minutes after consumption. Transmucosal fentanyl, which is frequently prescribed for breakthrough pain, is an exception to that statement. It is a nonintravenous full mu agonist with a rapid onset. Most SAOs, unless they are delivered intravenously, are absorbed slowly. In contrast, heroin that is smoked or inhaled has an onset of action of less than 1 minute, with a sharp peak followed by a rapid decline.

SAOs may, however, constitute a separate vulnerability to drug abuse because a short duration of action requires more frequent administration, which in turn may encourage the patient to binge to reach acceptable analgesia. The view that SAOs pose a greater risk of abuse than LAOs remains conjecture. LAOs that can be altered (eg, by crushing the pills) to release their sustained-action analgesia all at once could be considered more "abusable" than a shorter-duration opioid. This raises an important point: Often, experts on pain management and addiction are asked which drugs are most "abusable." Perhaps a more astute question would be, "Where is the genesis of abuse located: in the drug or in the individual who abuses it?" Although it is possible that research will establish an association between a particular drug and the patient's inability to control the consumption of that drug, it appears that addictive disease finds its locus in the individual rather than in the substance. Tsuang and colleagues, who studied polysubstance abuse, suggest there is "some characteristic of the individual that imparts vulnerability to the abuse of all categories of drugs."[8] The particular drug of abuse is probably far less important than the effect being sought. For that reason, abusers often vary the substances they abuse.

Although it is beneficial to consider the drug properties that could trigger the drug-abuse vulnerabilities of an individual who is predisposed to addiction, it should be remembered that a drug of abuse in the hands of one person is a godsend of pain relief to another. As medical science progresses, certain drugs can be expected to fall out of use when other drugs with greater effectiveness and better safety profiles become popular.

The Environment

We all live in and contribute to several different environments: family, work, community affairs, and social relationships. If, during our daily activities, we are exposed to the acceptance of substance abuse (be it alcohol, tobacco, marijuana or opiates), that exposure creates a vulnerability to drug abuse. Individuals who abuse drugs increase the likelihood that other people in the same environment will also abuse drugs. That influence can be seen in both in-home and out-of-home environments. Some of the vulnerability will be tied to the specific drug the individual observes being abused and some will not. For example, an environment that encourages marijuana consumption confers a strong vulnerability factor specific to marijuana that does not appear to extend to opioids. Yet for the most part, if any substance is abused within the family or among peers, the individual is at risk for abusing different categories of substances, not merely the one he or she observes being abused.

Peer Norms

Early drug use places children and adolescents on a dangerous track that all too frequently leads to drug abuse as adults. Children who use marijuana are 100 times more likely to use cocaine than are those who never use marijuana.[31] Research draws a direct parallel between peer approval of drug use and greater drug use (particularly first drug use) among adolescents. Whether the substance abuse continues or ceases is influenced by developmental factors and the presence of psychologic disorders, genetic vulnerability, and family dysfunction.

Factors related to adolescent drug abuse include:

• Poor self-image.
• Low religiosity.
• Poor school performance.
• Parental rejection.

• Family dysfunction.
• Child abuse.
• Undercontrolling or overcontrolling by parents.
• Parental divorce.[31]

Stress

The daily living conditions of a person who abuses drugs provide many situational and social cues that encourage continued drug misuse. One of those conditions is stress. In laboratory tests, rats exposed to the social stressor of a more aggressive rat learned to self-administer cocaine twice as fast as did nonstressed animals.[32]

Stress can exacerbate drug-abusing behavior in many ways.[33] Some stressful life events (the death of a loved one, divorce, a natural disaster, or a job loss) are isolated events. Other stressors (chronic health conditions, financial woes) are ongoing. The success with which people handle the stress in their lives varies as much as individuals do. We all know at least a few people whose lives resemble a never-ending train wreck; their problems are never solved but seem to multiply in an atmosphere of chaos and poor choices. Ongoing stress can worsen current abuse behaviors and can also precipitate a recurrence of substance abuse.[34]

Changes in life circumstances can create different propensities for abuse at different times in the same individual. This principle can be seen in laboratory experiments using inbred rats. Lewis rats self-administer more drugs than do Fischer-344 rats.[35] Sprague-Dawley rats are considered neither drug seeking nor drug rejecting but respond more like the drug-seeking rats if exposed to the right environmental or physiologic influences.[36] In rats,

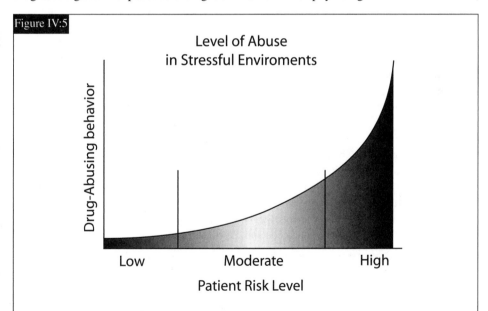

Figure IV:5

Level of Abuse in Stressful Enviroments

Drug-Abusing behavior

Low   Moderate   High

Patient Risk Level

Source: Webster LR. Determining the risk of opioid abuse. Emerging Solutions in Pain CE-Accredited Monograph. Practical Pain Management 2006 Jan-Feb; 6(1).

just as in humans, stress is one of the main stimuli that provokes drug-taking behavior.[37] Like rats, humans can be classified as being at high risk, moderate risk, or low risk for drug-seeking behavior. Stress can provoke abuse even in a person who otherwise would be unlikely to exhibit such behavior. Patients at moderate risk for drug abuse (the human equivalent of a Sprague-Dawley rat) demonstrate this concept most clearly. A person in the high-risk group may abuse drugs no matter what the circumstances, and a person at low risk for drug abuse is far less likely to do so, even when experiencing extraordinary stress. An individual at moderate risk may never abuse drugs under favorable or neutral life circumstances, but in a stressful environment (particularly if multiple stressors are present) where an abusable drug is available, he or she begins to behave more like an individual at high risk for substance abuse (Figure IV:5). The lesson for clinicians who prescribe opioids to treat pain is to understand the importance of assessing the patient's current life stressors to minimize the risk of opioid abuse. A patient may change risk categories for drug abuse more than once during a lifetime. This is especially true for people who occupy the middle of the risk spectrum.

Pain and Stress

Imagine the greatest physical pain you have experienced in your life, and then imagine that pain multiplied over weeks, months, and years with no end in sight. People who live with chronic pain live with pervasive stress, and their lives are forever changed. Pain is physically stressful. It interrupts sleep and disrupts hormone levels. Unremitting pain is also psychologically stressful. It causes low self-esteem and may result in loss of job or social standing. Financial worries may be overwhelming. Independence, mobility, and family relationships are compromised. There appears to be no escape from the merry-go-round of life lived in hospital emergency rooms. The chronic-pain patient is forever called on to justify his or her experience and to explain what is unexplainable. The possibility always looms that whatever pain relief is available will be snatched away because of the fear, misinformation, or apathy of the latest caregiver.

Taken together, these dynamics can lead patients to seek relief from the anxiety, depression, and boredom of a life lived in unremitting pain. The drive to escape — to chemically cope — is powerful and can lead to unauthorized escalations of prescription medication by patients. Oblivion can seem an attractive alternative to consciousness. People with chronic pain have high rates of attempted and completed suicides.[38]

Some healthcare professionals unwittingly add to their patients' stress. Healthcare providers are often advised erroneously to prescribe opioids in small quantities when a patient has trouble achieving adequate analgesia and begs for more medication. Clinicians are taught to suspect that patients who exceed some arbitrary ceiling dose of narcotic pain medications must be seeking opioids for personal misuse or sale. That attitude can cause great harm. If opioids have been determined to be the best treatment available for the individual in question, parsimonious prescribing is not the answer when pain is uncontrolled. The undertreatment of pain is poor medical practice and does not stop the spread of drug abuse.

Genetics

Genetics is known to exert an influence on drug abuse, but precisely which genes contribute to substance abuse and how they do so remains unknown. Studies comparing fraternal (nonidentical) twins with genetically identical twins are useful in assessing how genetics (as opposed to environment) influences the development of abuse behaviors. Studies highlighting outcomes of adopted children who are genetically vulnerable to substance abuse are also helpful. The research involving the genetic influence on substance abuse is best summarized thus: In general, it appears that an individual may begin using drugs experimentally because he or she is modeling behavior observed in social and family circles. If and when that behavior progresses to substance abuse or dependence, genetic factors are largely to blame[39] and exert a stronger influence on males than on females.[40]

As we have seen, genetic factors more greatly influence the abuse of some categories of drugs than others, and the role that environment plays can be hard to isolate. One area in which a genetic influence has been established involves alcohol abuse: The biological children of alcohol-dependent parents, even when adopted and raised in a nonalcoholic environment, demonstrate a 2-fold to 9-fold increased risk for alcohol abuse or dependence.[31] Cocaine and marijuana abuse and dependence (as distinguished from casual use) have also been linked to genetic factors; genetics was held responsible for 60% to 80% of the differences in abuse and dependence between fraternal and identical twin pairs. [39, 41]

Opioid Abuse

As noted earlier, it appears that a drug-abuse disorder involving opiates (including heroin and prescription opioids) may be driven by a strong genetic link. Emerging research indicates that the development of an addictive disorder involving opioids is about 50% determined by genetics.[8] A large study of male twin pairs found that the genetic influence on opiate abuse is specific primarily to opiate abuse and is not shared across categories of other drugs.[8] Although those researchers found little evidence that abuse of any specific drug "breeds true" within a particular family, the genetic link to multigenerational substance abuse, particularly for opiates, is well accepted among most experts.

Conclusion

Specific risk factors are linked to problematic drug use. For example, a personal or family history of substance abuse, a history of sexual abuse, and the presence of certain mental diseases all have proven useful in predicting whether a patient is likely to display aberrant behaviors consistent with abuse.[2] An individual's history, current life situation, and certain vulnerabilities such as stress, abuse-prone environments, the ingestion of a drug with binge potential, and a genetic predisposition can combine to form that individual's risk profile. A person's risk profile for drug abuse (except for genetically determined factors) may change over a lifetime. The more risk factors and vulnerabilities that are present, the greater the risk to the individual. The next chapter will present tools that can be used to assess a patient's level of risk.

References

1. Fitzhenry RI, ed. *The Harper Book of Quotations*. 3rd ed. New York, NY: Harper-Collins; 1993:283.
2. Webster LR, Webster RM. Predicting aberrant behaviors in opioid-treated patients: preliminary validation of the Opioid Risk Tool. Pain Med. 2005 Nov-Dec;6(6):432-42.

3. Savage SR. Assessment for addiction in pain-treatment settings. Clin J Pain. 2002 Jul-Aug;18(4 Suppl):S28-38.
4. Dunbar SA, Katz NP. Chronic opioid therapy for nonmalignant pain in patients with a history of substance abuse: report of 20 cases. J Pain Symptom Manage 1996; 11(3):163-171.
5. Friedman R, Li V, Mehrotra D. Treating pain patients at risk: evaluation of a screening tool in opioid-treated pain patients with and without addiction. Pain Med. 2003 Jun;4(2):182-5.
6. Atluri S, Sudarshan G. A screening tool to determine the risk of prescription opioid abuse among patients with chronic non-malignant pain [abstract]. Pain Physician. 2002; 5(4):447-48.
7. Chabal C, Erjavec MK, Jacobson L, Mariano A, Chaney E. Prescription opiate abuse in chronic pain patients: clinical criteria, incidence, and predictors. Clin J Pain. 1997 Jun;13(2):150-5.
8. Tsuang MT, Lyons MJ, Meyer JM, Doyle T, Eisen SA, Goldberg J, True W, Lin N, Toomey R, Eaves L. Co-occurrence of abuse of different drugs in men: the role of drug-specific and shared vulnerabilities. Arch Gen Psychiatry. 1998 Nov;55(11):967-72.
9. Regier DA, Farmer ME, Rae DS, Locke BZ, Keith SJ, Judd LL, Goodwin FK. Comorbidity of mental disorders with alcohol and other drug abuse. Results from the Epidemiologic Catchment Area (ECA) Study. JAMA. 1990 Nov 21;264(19):2511-8.
10. Staines GL, Magura S, Foote J, Deluca A, Kosanke N. Polysubstance use among alcoholics. J Addict Dis. 2001;20(4):53-69.
11. Meller WH, Rinehart R, Cadoret RJ, Troughton E. Specific familial transmission in substance abuse. Int J Addict. 1988 Oct;23(10):1029-39.
12. Merikangas KR, Stolar M, Stevens DE, Goulet J, Preisig MA, Fenton B, Zhang H, O'Malley SS, Rounsaville BJ. Familial transmission of substance use disorders. Arch Gen Psychiatry. 1998 Nov;55(11):973-9.
13. Prescott CA. Sex differences in the genetic risk for alcoholism. Alcohol Res Health. 2002;26(4):264-73.
14. Christie KA, Burke JD Jr, Regier DA, Rae DS, Boyd JH, Locke BZ. Epidemiologic evidence for early onset of mental disorders and higher risk of drug abuse in young adults. Am J Psychiatry. 1988 Aug;145(8):971-5.
15. Ross HE, Glaser FB, Germanson T. The prevalence of psychiatric disorders in patients with alcohol and other drug problems. Arch Gen Psychiatry. 1988 Nov;45(11):1023-31.
16. Buntin-Mushock C, Phillip L, Moriyama K, Palmer PP. Age-dependent opioid escalation in chronic pain patients. Anesth Analg. 2005 Jun;100(6):1740-5.
17. Swan N. Exploring the role of child abuse in later drug abuse. NIDA Notes 1998; 13(2).
18. Kendler KS, Bulik CM, Silberg J, Hettema JM, Myers J, Prescott CA. Childhood sexual abuse and adult psychiatric and substance use disorders in women: an epidemiological and cotwin control analysis. Arch Gen Psychiatry. 2000 Oct;57(10):953-9.

19. Bifulco A, Brown GW, Adler Z. Early sexual abuse and clinical depression in adult life. Br J Psychiatry. 1991 Jul;159:115-22.
20. Najavits LM, Weiss RD, Shaw SR. The link between substance abuse and post-traumatic stress disorder in women. A research review. Am J Addict. 1997 Fall;6(4):273-83.
21. Yehuda R. Post-traumatic stress disorder. New Engl J Med 2002;346(2):1495-8.
22. Kessler RC, Chiu WT, Demler O, Merikangas KR, Walters EE. Prevalence, severity, and comorbidity of 12-month DSM-IV disorders in the National Comorbidity Survey Replication. Arch Gen Psychiatry. 2005 Jun;62(6):617-27. Erratum in: Arch Gen Psychiatry. 2005 Jul;62(7):709. Merikangas, Kathleen R.
23. Kessler RC, Berglund P, Demler O, Jin R, Merikangas KR, Walters EE. Lifetime prevalence and age-of-onset distributions of DSM-IV disorders in the National Comorbidity Survey Replication. Arch Gen Psychiatry. 2005 Jun;62(6):593-602. Erratum in: Arch Gen Psychiatry. 2005 Jul;62(7):768. Merikangas, Kathleen R.
24. Volkow ND. The dual challenge of substance abuse and mental disorders. NIDA Notes. 2003; 18(5):3-4.
25. Farrell M, Howes S, Bebbington P, Brugha T, Jenkins R, Lewis G, Marsden J, Taylor C, Meltzer H. Nicotine, alcohol and drug dependence, and psychiatric comorbidity—results of a national household survey. Int Rev Psychiatry. 2003 Feb-May;15(1-2):50-6.
26. Biederman J, Wilens T, Mick E, Spencer T, Faraone SV. Pharmacotherapy of attention-deficit/hyperactivity disorder reduces risk for substance use disorder. Pediatrics. 1999 Aug;104(2):e20.
27. Brady KT, Grice DE, Dustan L, Randall C. Gender differences in substance use disorders. Am J Psychiatry. 1993 Nov;150(11):1707-11.
28. Swan N. Gender affects relationships between drug abuse and psychiatric disorders. NIDA Notes 1997; 12(4).
29. Studies show wide range of co-occurring disorders. Substance Abuse Newsletter., Pace Publications. 2003; 9:5.
30. Rosenblum A, Joseph H, Fong C, Kipnis S, Cleland C, Portenoy RK. Prevalence and characteristics of chronic pain among chemically dependent patients in methadone maintenance and residential treatment facilities. JAMA. 2003 May 14;289(18):2370-8.
31. Belcher HM, Shinitzky HE. Substance abuse in children: prediction, protection, and prevention. Arch Pediatr Adolesc Med. 1998 Oct;152(10):952-60.
32. Bowersox JA. Anxiety and stress found to promote cocaine use in rats. NIDA Notes 1996; 11(4).
33. Piazza PV, Le Moal M. The role of stress in drug self-administration. Trends Pharmacol Sci. 1998 Feb;19(2):67-74.
34. Koob GF, Le Moal M. Drug abuse: hedonic homeostatic dysregulation. Science. 1997 Oct 3;278(5335):52-8.
35. Gosnell BA, Krahn DD. Morphine-induced feeding: a comparison of the Lewis and Fischer 344 inbred rat strains. Pharmacol Biochem Behav. 1993 Apr;44(4):919-24.

36. Kabbaj M, Norton CS, Kollack-Walker S, Watson SJ, Robinson TE, Akil H. Social defeat alters the acquisition of cocaine self-administration in rats: role of individual differences in cocaine-taking behavior. Psychopharmacology (Berl). 2001 Dec;158(4):382-7. Epub 2001 Nov 1.

37. Gardner EL. What we have learned about addiction from animal models of drug self-administration. Am J Addict. 2000 Fall;9(4):285-313.

38. Fishbain DA. The association of chronic pain and suicide. Semin Clin Neuropsychiatry. 1999 Jul;4(3):221-7.

39. Kendler KS, Prescott CA. Cocaine use, abuse and dependence in a population-based sample of female twins. Br J Psychiatry. 1998 Oct;173:345-50.

40. van den Bree MB, Johnson EO, Neale MC, Pickens RW. Genetic and environmental influences on drug use and abuse/dependence in male and female twins. Drug Alcohol Depend. 1998 Nov 1;52(3):231-41.

41. Kendler KS, Prescott CA. Cannabis use, abuse, and dependence in a population-based sample of female twins. Am J Psychiatry. 1998 Aug;155(8):1016-22.

CHAPTER V

ASSESSING PATIENTS FOR THE RISK OF OPIOID ABUSE

He who asks is a fool for five minutes, but he who does not ask remains a fool forever.
- Chinese Proverb

A patient's probability of opioid abuse is linked to certain risk factors that are influenced by genetics and environment. Knowing whether a patient exhibits risk factors before the initiation of treatment enables clinicians to set the appropriate level of monitoring, which in turn helps to prevent abuse. Therefore, all patients who are to begin treatment with long-term opioid therapy for pain must undergo assessment for potential drug abuse. Patients usually fall into 1 of 3 groups with respect to their potential for abusing drugs: low risk, moderate risk, or high risk. The higher the degree of risk, the more stringent the required monitoring. The purpose of classifying patients into risk categories is not to isolate high-risk patients and deny them the pain treatment they need but to increase the likelihood of a good clinical outcome for all patients.

This chapter identifies and evaluates the most common assessments used to screen for existing or potential substance abuse. Emphasis is placed on the need for methods of assessment that are brief, opioid specific, easy to administer and interpret, and consistent in providing results.

Screening Can Prevent Abuse

Although the misuse of medication is a common clinical occurrence, it is manageable in most cases. The vital first step is the appropriate assessment of the patient before opioid therapy is initiated. Armed with the results of that assessment, clinicians can use a scientific approach based on the patient's level of risk for substance abuse to monitor a patient's opioid consumption. The practice of screening patients who begin opioid therapy for potential problematic drug behavior is in its infancy.[1] However, research to support the practice of assessment is increasing every day. Despite studies showing that systematic screening is the best tool for discerning current and lifetime substance-use disorders, such screening is often not performed. One study showed that primary care and behavioral health clinicians failed to detect substance problems in more than 80% of cases in which the patient had clearly checked items related to substance abuse on a questionnaire.[2] Primary care physicians and other healthcare professionals can make a vital contribution to recognizing and treating substance-use disorders. About 70% of Americans visit their primary care physician at least once every 2 years.[3] Furthermore, chronic-pain patients are significant consumers of primary care medical services, which they use up to 5 times more frequently than do other patients.[4] Patient assessment is not performed for a number of reasons. A survey of 2000 general physicians and psychiatrists identified some of the barriers that healthcare providers face in screening patients for substance abuse:

• Lack of confidence in addiction-management capabilities.
• Perception of time limitations.
• Fears about patient sensitivity surrounding substance-abuse issues.[5]

   These concerns are understandable but surmountable, given the proper tools and training. It is important that clinicians not be dissuaded from discussing the potential for substance abuse with their patients.

Criteria for the Assessment of Substance Abuse by Patients

   Physicians and other clinicians without training in addiction medicine would be greatly helped by the wider availability of proven tools for assessing substance abuse in their patients. To be useful in a busy medical practice, those assessment tools must be:

• *Predictive*. Assessments that detect current substance abuse are helpful but do not provide for the establishment of a suitable level of monitoring before the initiation of opioid therapy.
• *Brief.* Time limitations on office visits dictate the need for a brief assessment. Longer assessments are impractical for many clinicians and may lead to nonuse of the instrument.
• *Easy to administer and interpret*. The need for special training to score and interpret results does not meet the requirement for widespread clinical utility.
• *Geared to opioid abuse rather than the abuse of alcohol or other substances*. Screening all patients for general substance abuse is an advisable part of medical practice. However, patients who suffer from chronic pain and who are being considered as candidates for long-term opioid therapy present a more specific need for drug assessment.
• *Validated in patients with pain*. The assessment should be validated for use in chronic-pain patients who are being considered for long-term opioid therapy.
• *Applicable to a variety of clinical settings*. Little is known about the differences between chronic-pain patients treated in primary care practices and those treated in pain clinics. Because patients in pain are treated in a variety of settings, the best type of assessment would apply in a variety of pain-patient populations.
• *Self-administered*. A self-administered tool may save time and clinical resources, which would render its use likely.

   Most of the assessments available contain some but not all of these attributes. Each tool has unique advantages and disadvantages, as the following discussion reveals.

Limitations of Familiar Screening Tools

   Many of the tools available for use in screening for prescription opioid abuse do not yet meet the needs of patients and clinicians. Of the currently available modalities used to screen patients for substance abuse, many exhibit 1 or more of the following common problems:

• They are designed to identify patients who already have problems with managing substance intake and not to predict those who may abuse drugs.

• They are not designed to screen specifically for opioid abuse.
• They take a long time to administer and require unique skills to interpret.

Research is beginning to address some of those concerns. Efforts are under way to design assessments (derived from the literature or expert opinion) that address the specific needs of opioid-treated pain patients. Meanwhile, a number of already available screening tools provide some clinical utility, although clinicians should be aware of their inadequacies with respect to evaluating chronic-pain patients.

Characteristics of Common Assessments: A Comparison

Some of the available substance-abuse screening tools, old and new, are listed in Box V:1, which illustrates at a glance whether specific assessments are:

• Specific to alcohol, nonalcoholic drugs, or both.
• Predictive of subsequent abuse problems.
• Validated in the population of interest (in this case, pain patients).
• Self-administered.
• Brief to perform.

Diagnostic Versus Screening Tools

Most screening tools are not designed to diagnose substance-use disorders. If patients demonstrate a positive score from screening for substance abuse, they should be considered candidates for an additional evaluation to diagnose whether an actual substance-use disorder is present. Many diagnostic tools are rather cumbersome to administer and score and are not intended for initial screening for substance abuse.

One of these is the Structured Clinical Interview,[6] which is a thorough assessment that is widely used by research centers and substance-abuse treatment centers staffed by professionals who are trained to administer and score it. Another tool that is especially effective for evaluating the need for substance-abuse treatment is the Addiction Severity Index,[7] a 200-item hour-long assessment of 7 potential problem areas, which is designed to be administered by a trained interviewer. Those 2 assessments are valuable for evaluating many psychiatric, social, and substance problems, but their length and the special training required for their use render them impractical for widespread clinical use. In contrast, brief screening tools are less cumbersome to administer. However, they are usually designed to identify patients who already have problems with substances rather than to predict those who may abuse drugs. Two examples of such assessments are the widely used alcohol-specific CAGE test ("cut, annoyed, guilty, eye")[8] and another tool called the Two-Item Conjoint Screen (TICS),[9] which is a 2-question measure of sensitivity to substance abuse. Those instruments are not intended for use in screening specifically for opioid abuse, although in some cases they can be modified for such use. They could have some clinical utility in the field of chronic pain, because individuals who are addicted to alcohol or another drug are at increased risk for abusing opioids.

Tools Specific for the Assessment of Alcohol Abuse

Alcohol-related disorders have been the subject of much research, so it is not surprising to find that some of the most widely validated screeners and assessments are specific

| Box V:1 | | | | Tests for Identifying Potential Drug Abuse | |

Tool	Alcohol/ Drugs	Predictive of Substance Abuse	Pain Patients	Method of Test Administration	Length of Test and Time Required for Completion
Addiction Severity Index	Yes/Yes	No	No	Self and/or interview	200 items 1 h
Alcohol Use Disorders Identification Test	Yes/No	No	No	Self and/or interview	10 items 2 min
Structured Clinical Interview for *DSM-IV* (psychoactive substance use module only)	Yes/Yes	Yes	No	Interview	30-60 min
CAGE	Yes/No	No	No	Interview	4 items < 1 min
CAGE-Adapted to Include Drugs	Yes/Yes	No	No	Interview	4 items < 1 min
Two-Item Conjoint Screening Tool	Yes/Yes	No	No	Interview	2 items < 1 min
Screener and Opioid Assessment for Patients with Pain	Yes/Yes	Yes	Yes	Self and/or interview	24 items 10 min
Prescription Drug Use Questionnaire	Yes/Yes	Yes	Yes	Interview	42 items 20 min
RAFFT	Yes/Yes	No	No	Self	5 items About 1 min
Drug Abuse Screening Test	No/Yes	No	No	Self	20 items 5 min
Michigan Alcohol Screening Test	Yes/No	No	No	Self and/or interview	Long version: 25 items 15 min Short versions: 9 to 13 items
Screening Instrument for Substance Abuse Potential	Yes/Yes	Yes	No	Interview	5 items About 1 min
Substance Abuse Subtle Screening Inventory-3	Yes/Yes	No	No	Self	1 page 15 min
Severity of Opiate Dependence Questionnaire	No/Yes	No	No	Self	21 items About 5 min
Opioid Risk Tool	Yes/Yes	Yes	Yes	Self	5 items 1 min

for alcohol abuse. Although the following assessments have not been validated among pain patients and do not address the risk factors specific to opioid abuse, they are sometimes used to assess for opioid abuse.

CAGE.[8] This 4-item verbal test has been validated in several studies as an effective screening for the identification of lifetime alcohol-abuse disorders. Two affirmative answers are considered a positive result from screening, although many clinicians consider even 1 affirmative reply cause for concern. The CAGE was later adapted to include other types of drug abuse in addition to alcohol. For opioid-treated patients, it might be beneficial to consider adapting the CAGE to invite open-ended answers rather than "yes/no" responses (ie, "how often have you ...").

Michigan Alcoholism Screening Test (MAST).[10] Long and short versions of the MAST are available. The long version has 25 items, and the shorter versions contains 10 to 13 items. The MAST is one of the first alcohol screening tests and one of the most widely used. It is particularly useful for assessing lifetime problems with alcohol abuse. Its accuracy rates are similar to those of the CAGE, though it takes longer to administer. A still longer 37-item test called the Self-Administered Alcoholism Screening Test[11] has been derived from the MAST. An evaluation is under way to add a screening component for other drugs to the MAST.

Alcohol Use Disorders Identification Test[12]. This is a 10-item written test available through the World Health Organization to identify harmful alcohol consumption in many populations, including patients treated in primary care practices, psychiatric units, and prisons. However, because it is self-administered and takes longer than some other similar evaluations, it is less popular with clinicians than are quick verbal assessments, such as the CAGE.

In an evaluation of alcohol screening tools, the Alcohol Use Disorders Identification Test was found to be most effective in identifying subjects at risk for harmful drinking, and the CAGE was superior in detecting alcohol abuse and dependence.[13]

Conjoint Screening Tools

Several instruments have been created or adapted to screen simultaneously and with the same question for alcohol and other drug abuse. The advantages of a conjoint screening tool are to save time and to encourage a patient to answer more honestly than he or she might when responding to separate questions. However, people who abuse only alcohol may answer with a negative response because they want to avoid appearing to abuse illicit or prescription drugs. Two of the briefer tools that fall into this category are the CAGE-Adapted to Include Drugs (CAGE-AID)[14] (Box V:2) and the TICS[9] (Box V:3). The sensitivity and specificity of the CAGE-AID, which are shown in the corresponding Box, are still high, though the specificity is less than that of the alcohol-specific CAGE.

The TICS is said to identify 80% of drug and alcohol problems in young and middle-age patients by asking 2 easily remembered questions. This evaluation is brief and easy to administer. However, the CAGE-AID and the TICS are not opioid specific and are designed to detect current and lifelong substance abuse, not to assess the risk of future abuse.

Tools for Identifying Drug Abuse in Patients

Modeled on the MAST, the self-administered Drug Abuse Screening Test[15] (Box V:4) contains many items that can be used to identify problems caused by drug abuse other than

---

Box V:2

The CAGE-Adapted to Include Drugs Questionnaire

In the past have you ever:

1. Tried to cut down or change your pattern of drinking or drug abuse?
2. Been annoyed or angry by others' concern about your drinking or drug use?
3. Felt guilty about the consequences of your drinking or drug use?
4. Had a drink or used a drug in the morning (an "eye-opener") to decrease a hangover or withdrawal symptoms?

Implications for prescribing:

- One positive response to any question suggests caution.
- Two or more positive responses may have a sensitivity of 60% to 95% and a specificity of 40% to 95% for diagnosing alcohol or drug problems. Strongly suggest assessment by an addiction specialist before opioids are prescribed.
- A CAGE test result may have less predictive value in the elderly, college students, women, and certain ethnic groups.

---

alcohol. Some of the problems it addresses include drug-related blackouts, job-related problems, and social and family discord. It also contains a specific item used to screen for prescription drug abuse. The DAST is brief and can be administered without special training. It is valuable for determining which patients should seek substance-abuse treatment but has not been validated for use in pain patients. Like the MAST, it has been suggested that the DAST is focused primarily on problems with employment, violence, and illegal activities, and its lack of questions about home and children make it more applicable to men than women. The RAFFT[16] ("relax, alone, friends, family, trouble") (Box V:5) is a 5-question screening tool that is used to detect alcohol and drug abuse and has performed well in adolescents. It is brief and easy to score. However, in a study of adult psychiatric patients, it was reported to be less specific than in adolescents.[16]

The Substance Abuse Subtle Screening Inventory (SASSI)[17] is a widely used instrument that is available from the SASSI Institute in Bloomington, Indiana. This 1-page questionnaire combines face-valid questions with subtle questions that do not address substance

---

Box V:3

TICS: A Two-Item Conjoint Screen

1) In the last year, have you ever drunk or used drugs more than you meant to?
2) Have you felt you wanted or needed to cut down on your drinking or drug use in the last year?

In primary care patients, at least 1 affirmative answer to these 2 questions was nearly 80% sensitive and specific for substance abuse.

Box V:4

The Drug Abuse Screening Test (DAST)

The following questions concern information about your involvement and abuse of drugs. "Drug abuse" refers to:

(1) The use of prescribed or over-the-counter drugs in excess of directions.

(2) Any nonmedical use of drugs.

The questions DO NOT include alcoholic beverages.

The questions refer to the past 12 months. Carefully read each statement and decide whether your answer is "yes" or "no." Please give the best answer or the answer that is right most of the time. Click on the box marked "Yes" or "No."

1. Have you used drugs other than those required for medical reasons?	Yes / No
2. Have you abused prescription drugs?	Yes / No
3. Do you abuse more than 1 drug at a time?	Yes / No
4. Can you get through the week without using drugs?	Yes / No
5. Are you always able to stop using drugs when you want to?	Yes / No
6. Have you had "blackouts" or "flashbacks" as a result of drug use?	Yes / No
7. Do you ever feel bad or guilty about your drug use?	Yes / No
8. Does your spouse (or do your parents) ever complain about your involvement with drugs?	Yes / No
9. Has drug abuse created problems between you and your spouse or your parents?	Yes / No
10. Have you lost friends because of your use of drugs?	Yes / No
11. Have you neglected your family because of your use of drugs?	Yes / No
12. Have you been in trouble at work because of your use of drugs?	Yes / No
13. Have you lost a job because of drug abuse?	Yes / No
14. Have you gotten into fights when you were under the influence of drugs?	Yes / No
15. Have you engaged in illegal activities to obtain drugs?	Yes / No
16. Have you been arrested for possession of illegal drugs?	Yes / No
17. Have you ever experienced withdrawal symptoms (felt sick) when you stopped taking drugs?	Yes / No
18. Have you had medical problems as a result of your drug use (eg, memory loss, hepatitis, convulsions, bleeding, etc)?	Yes / No
19. Have you gone to anyone for help for a drug problem?	Yes / No
20. Have you been involved in a treatment program especially related to drug use?	Yes / No

---

Box V:5   **RAFFT ("relax, alone, friends, family, trouble")**

Relax: Do you drink/drug to relax, feel better about yourself, or fit in?

Alone: Do you ever drink/drug while you are by yourself (alone)?

Friends: Do any of your closest friends drink/drug?

Family: Does a close family member have a problem with alcohol/drugs?

Trouble: Have you ever gotten into trouble from drinking/drugging?

Three affirmative responses constitute a positive score. This test produced more false-positive results in adults than in adolescents.

---

abuse directly. The intent is to circumvent a presumed reluctance on the part of the subject to speak frankly about substance abuse. The primary use of the SASSI is to plan for treatment in a variety of criminal justice, mental health, vocational, educational, and other settings. The revised SASSI-3 demonstrated a 95% agreement with diagnoses of substance dependence in a range of clinical settings. The SASSI is also available in a format geared to adolescents.

The Severity of Opiate Dependence Questionnaire[18] (Box V:6), which has been validated in English and Australian heroin users, is intended for use as a measure of opiate dependence, not as an initial screening for opioid-treated pain patients. The multiple-choice questions have been divided into 5 sections that address patterns of drug abuse, the degree of withdrawal symptoms, and other signs of physical and psychologic dependence on substances of abuse. The Severity of Opiate Dependence Questionnaire is used to measure signs of addiction, including whether there is an increased focus on obtaining the substance, whether the patient is aware of his or her compulsion to abuse drugs, and the patient's inability to stop abusing the drug of choice, even after a period of abstinence. Its specificity to opiates is an advantage, although it may not address disparities between users of illegal street drugs and prescription drug abusers. No cutoff score has been established, and clinical judgment must be used to evaluate the patient's test answers to determine whether he or she is opiate dependent.

A New Generation of Opioid-Specific Tools

One thing should be clear from the preceding brief overview of the most widely available tools: Although they are clinically useful, the available tools have not yet been tailored to the specific needs of opioid-treated pain patients. That is beginning to change. A number of new tools used to screen for and assess the risk of prescription-drug abuse have recently been made available. They include questions related to mental disorders, past sexual abuse, and lifestyle factors and are designed to help clinicians isolate and even predict medication misuse in patients with pain. These newer tools have been shown to be valid in limited clinical trials, although more research is needed to demonstrate their applicability to broader patient populations. A discussion of these tools with supporting documentation follows.

The Prescription Drug Use Questionnaire

The promising new batch of opioid-specific assessments includes the 42-item Prescription Drug Use Questionnaire[19] (PDUQ) (Box V:7). This interview to be administered by the clinician collects a wealth of data detailing the patient's painful condition, opioid use, social and family factors, and psychiatric history. In a pilot study,[19] scores from 6 to 15 were recorded for nonaddicted subjects, from 11 to 25 for substance-abusing subjects, and from 15 to 28 for substance-dependent subjects. All subjects whose score was higher than 15 later satisfied the criteria for a substance-use disorder; therefore, the questionnaire appears to have some predictive validity. However, the PDUQ takes longer to administer than is practical in many clinical situations.

The Opioid Risk Tool

A brief assessment for opioid abuse that has been validated in initial clinical tests is the first author's Opioid Risk Tool[20] (ORT) (Box V:8). The ORT is a 5-question self-administered assessment that takes fewer than 5 minutes to complete. In preliminary trials,[20] the ORT accurately predicted which patients were at highest and lowest risk for displaying aberrant drug-related behaviors (eg, using more opioids than prescribed, selling prescriptions, losing prescriptions or reporting them stolen, canceling clinic visits, forging prescriptions) associated with abuse or addiction. Designed for use during the initial visit for pain treatment, the ORT assesses the patient's personal and family history of prescription, alcohol, and illegal drug abuse; age; history of preadolescent sexual abuse; and the presence of depression, attention deficit disorder, obsessive-compulsive disorder, bipolar disorder, or schizophrenia. The selection of these items was based on a review of the scientific literature that showed their value in predicting the later development of a substance-use disorder.

In that study,[20] 185 new patients who were receiving opioids to treat chronic pain took the ORT during their initial visit. They were grouped according to their ORT scores into categories of high, moderate, or low risk and were then monitored for 12 months. Of the low-risk patients, 17 of 18 (94.4%) did not display an aberrant behavior. Of the high-risk patients, 40 of 44 (90.9%) did display an aberrant behavior.

The ORT represents a move toward addressing the need to predict who is at risk for opioid abuse before opioid therapy is initiated. This gives physicians a better opportunity to monitor moderate-to-high-risk patients rather than waiting until after treatment has begun to check for abuse.

The Screener and Opioid Assessment for Patients with Pain (SOAPP)

Another relatively brief, recently validated assessment is the Screener and Opioid Assessment for Patients with Pain[21] (SOAPP) (Box V:9). The SOAPP is a 24-item self-assessment questionnaire that takes about 10 minutes to complete. It is intended for use only by chronic-pain patients who are being considered for long-term opioid therapy. In one study,[21] 154 patients who were taking opioids for chronic pain took the SOAPP. Six months later, 91 of the patients again completed the SOAPP and were also evaluated via the PDUQ, urine drug tests, and staff observation for medication misuse. Sixteen of the 24 questions in the SOAPP were found to predict aberrant behavior during the 6 months that followed the initial assessment. A score of 7 or higher was considered positive for the likelihood to abuse. More recent preliminary validation data divided patients into high-risk and low-risk categories using a cutoff score of 8.[22] Patients in the high-risk group were more likely to have an abnormal result from urine screening than were those in the low-risk group ($P < .05$), and patients with urine screening results in their medical chart had higher SOAPP scores than did patients who did not ($P < .001$).[22]

| Box V-6 | Severity of Opiate Dependence Questionnaire (SODQ) |

NAME_____AGE_____SEX_____

First of all, we would like you to recall a month when you were using opiates heavily in a way that, for you, was fairly typical of a heavy-use period. Please fill in the month and the year.

MONTH_____YEAR_____

Answer every question by circling 1 response only.
1. **On waking, and before my first dose of opiates**
   a. My body feels stiff:
   NEVER, SOMETIMES, OFTEN, ALWAYS,
   ALMOST NEVER, NEARLY ALWAYS
   b. I get stomach cramps:
   NEVER, SOMETIMES, OFTEN, ALWAYS,
   ALMOST NEVER, NEARLY ALWAYS
   c. I feel sick:
   NEVER, SOMETIMES, OFTEN, ALWAYS,
   ALMOST NEVER, NEARLY ALWAYS
   d. I notice my heart pounding:
   NEVER, SOMETIMES, OFTEN, ALWAYS,
   ALMOST NEVER, NEARLY ALWAYS
   e. I have hot and cold flashes:
   NEVER, SOMETIMES, OFTEN, ALWAYS,
   ALMOST NEVER, NEARLY ALWAYS
   f. I feel miserable or depressed:
   NEVER, SOMETIMES, OFTEN, ALWAYS,
   ALMOST NEVER, NEARLY ALWAYS
   g. I feel tense or panicky:
   NEVER, SOMETIMES, OFTEN, ALWAYS,
   ALMOST NEVER, NEARLY ALWAYS
   h. I feel irritable or angry:
   NEVER, SOMETIMES, OFTEN, ALWAYS,
   ALMOST NEVER, NEARLY ALWAYS
   i. I feel restless or unable to relax:
   NEVER, SOMETIMES, OFTEN, ALWAYS,
   ALMOST NEVER, NEARLY ALWAYS
   j. I have a strong craving:
   NEVER, SOMETIMES, OFTEN, ALWAYS,
   ALMOST NEVER, NEARLY ALWAYS

2. **Please complete all sections (a-f) of this question:**
   a. I try to save some opiates to use on waking:
   NEVER, SOMETIMES, OFTEN, ALWAYS,
   ALMOST NEVER, NEARLY ALWAYS
   b. I like to take my first dose of opiates within 2 hours of waking up:
   NEVER, SOMETIMES, OFTEN, ALWAYS,
   ALMOST NEVER, NEARLY ALWAYS
   c. In the morning, I use opiates to stop myself feeling sick:
   NEVER, SOMETIMES, OFTEN, ALWAYS,
   ALMOST NEVER, NEARLY ALWAYS
   d. The first thing I feel like doing when I wake up is to take some opiates:
   NEVER, SOMETIMES, OFTEN, ALWAYS,
   ALMOST NEVER, NEARLY ALWAYS
   e. When I wake up, I take opiates to stop myself aching or feeling stiff:
   NEVER, SOMETIMES, OFTEN, ALWAYS,
   ALMOST NEVER, NEARLY ALWAYS
   f. The first thing I do after waking up is to take some opiates:
   NEVER, SOMETIMES, OFTEN, ALWAYS,
   ALMOST NEVER, NEARLY ALWAYS

3. **Please think of your opiate use during a typical period of drug taking for these questions:**
   a. Did you think your opiate use was out of control?
   NEVER, SOMETIMES, OFTEN, ALWAYS,
   ALMOST NEVER, NEARLY ALWAYS
   b. Did the prospect of missing a fix (or dose) make you very anxious or worried?
   NEVER, SOMETIMES, OFTEN, ALWAYS,
   ALMOST NEVER, NEARLY ALWAYS
   c. Did you worry about your opiate use?
   NEVER, SOMETIMES, OFTEN, ALWAYS,
   ALMOST NEVER, NEARLY ALWAYS
   d. Did you wish you could stop?
   NEVER, SOMETIMES, OFTEN, ALWAYS,
   ALMOST NEVER, NEARLY ALWAYS
   e. How difficult would you find it to stop or go without?
   IMPOSSIBLE, VERY, QUITE, NOT DIFFICULT

Scoring
Answers to each question are rated on a 4-point scale. A score indicative of dependence has not yet been developed.

Box V-7	Prescription Drug Use Questionnaire:

Answer "yes" or "no"
Evaluation of the Pain Condition:

1. Does the patient have more than one painful condition (i.e., chronic back pain complicated by acute migraines or frequent dental work)?
2. Is the patient disabled by pain (i.e., unable to complete social or vocational activities of daily living)?
3. Is the patient receiving disability (i.e., SSI, worker comp.)?
4. Is the patient involved in litigation around the pain-precipitating incident?
5. Has the patient explored and/or tried nonopioid or nonpharmacological pain management techniques (i.e., physical therapy, TENS unit, relaxation, biofeedback) to manage pain?
6. Does the patient believe that his/her pain has been adequately treated over the past 6 months?
7. Does the patient express anger/mistrust of past health care providers?
8. Does the patient believe that he/she is addicted to opioid analgesics?
9. Does the referring physician believe that the patient is addicted to opioid analgesics?

Opioid Use Patterns:

9a. How long has the patient been on continuous opioids? (months)
10. Does the patient have more than one prescription provider (including dentists, ER physicians)?
11. Is there a pattern of the patient increasing prescribed analgesic dose or frequency?
12. Is there a pattern of the patient calling in for early prescription refills?
13. Does the patient report using analgesics for symptoms other than those prescribed for (i.e., insomnia, anxiety, depression)?
14. Does the patient save/hoard unused medication or have partially unused bottles of medication at home?
15. Does the patient report supplementing analgesics with alcohol or other psychoactive drugs (i.e., Soma, benzodiazepines)?
15a. If yes, please list:
16. Has the patient ever forged a prescription?
17. Is there a pattern of the patient reporting losing his/her medication?
18. Does the patient have preferences for specific analgesics and/or routes of administration (i.e, IV, IM routes over oral)?
19. Is there a pattern of the patient making emergency room visits for analgesics?
20. Has the patient ever obtained analgesic from nonmedical (street) sources?
21. Has any M.D./D.D.S. limited care, expressed concern, or refused to prescribe opioid analgesics because of patient's opioid use patterns?

Social/Family Factors:

22. Have family members expressed concern that the patient is addicted?
23. Are family members concerned about opioid analgesic side effects or tolerance?
24. Is there a pattern of family interaction that sustains the patient's opioid analgesic use? (i.e., family member overly concerned re: pain or withdrawal)
25. Is there a pattern of family interaction that sustains the patient's illness behavior or pain symptoms? (i.e, family member assuming caretaker role)
26. Does the spouse/significant other have a history of alcoholism/drug abuse/drug misuse?
27. Has a family member or friend ever obtained analgesic for the patient?
28. Has the patient ever taken analgesics prescribed for a friend or family member?
29. Does a family member or friend have access (either legal or illegal) to opioid analgesics (i.e., a family member in the medical profession)

Family History:
30. Is there a positive history of addiction (to any drug including alcohol) in the patient's mother, father, sibling or blood relative?
31. Is there a positive family history of chronic pain in the patient's mother, father, sibling or blood relative?

Patient History of Substance Abuse:

32. Did intoxication play a role in pain-precipitating incident?
33. Has the patient ever been diagnosed with addiction to any drug or alcohol?
34. Does the patient have a drug or alcohol treatment history?
35. Has opioid analgesic detoxification been previously attempted?
Psychiatric History:
36. Has the patient ever been diagnosed with a psychiatric disorder?
37. Did psychiatric symptoms precede onset of pain?
38. Is there a large psychological component to the pain condition, other than those related to addiction (i.e., multiple psychological stressors)
39. Is there evidence of a somatoform disorder?
40. Does the patient report a history of sexual or physical abuse?
41. Does the patient currently meet DSM-IV criteria for any Axis I, II or III conditions?
41a. If so, please list diagnoses:
42. Please list all pain-producing medical conditions:

Box V:8

Opioid Risk Tool

Item	Mark each box that applies	Item score if female	Item score if male
1. Family history of substance abuse			
Alcohol	[ ]	1	3
Illegal drugs	[ ]	2	3
Prescription drugs	[ ]	4	4
2. Personal history of substance abuse			
Alcohol	[ ]	3	3
Illegal drugs	[ ]	4	4
Prescription drugs	[ ]	5	5
3. Age (mark box if 16-45)	[ ]	1	1
4. History of preadolescent sexual abuse	[ ]	3	0
5. Psychologic disease			
Attention deficit disorder, obsessive-compulsive disorder, bipolar disorder, schizophrenia	[ ]	2	2
Depression	[ ]	1	1
Total		____	____
Total score risk category: Low risk: Zero - 3 Moderate risk: 4 - 7 High risk: 8 or higher			

The SOAPP questions were developed by a panel of pain experts. Like the ORT, the SOAPP was designed specifically to help clinicians make decisions about the level of monitoring needed by their patients receiving opioid treatment. Information from the SOAPP Web site[23] proclaims the test's reliability and reasonable predictive validity but also stresses the requirement for ongoing tests. Recent tweaking of the SOAPP has produced 2 additional versions: One contains 14 questions, and the shorter form contains 5 questions.

The shorter form, which has a cutoff score of 4, is a bit less accurate than the longer forms, which the researchers posit as a tradeoff that might be acceptable, given the savings in time when the short form is used. The 14-question SOAPP appears to have a sensitivity and specificity comparable to those of the original SOAPP 1.0.

The Screening Instrument for Substance Abuse Potential

Another tool that should be mentioned is the Screening Instrument for Substance Abuse Potential[24] (SISAP) (Box V:10). This assessment is a 5-item screen that is intended to help clinicians assess patients' risk for abusing opioids according to alcohol consumption, marijuana use, cigarette use, and age. Tested against a large database of nearly 5000 telephone survey responses in a Canadian epidemiologic survey of alcohol and drug use, the SISAP correctly classified 91% of substance abusers and 78% of nonabusers.[24] The instrument netted very few false–negative results but did have a high false-positive rate; 18% of the subjects were incorrectly identified as substance abusers. The SISAP has not been prospectively validated in a chronic-pain population, nor has it proven useful as yet in clinical settings.

Accuracy of Assessment Tools

To be valuable in a clinical setting, a screening tool should be both reliable and valid according to the cutoff score or scores chosen. A reliable tool yields repeatable and consistent results in a variety of applications. Validity is an indication that the tool measures what it is intended to measure. Sensitivity and specificity are 2 measures that indicate how valid a given assessment is within the population tested.

Sensitivity and Specificity

"Sensitivity" is the proportion of times that a positive score detects a true positive; ie, the percentage of subjects who test positive and who go on to display the measure's criteria for a substance-use disorder or an aberrant behavior that indicates possible abuse. "Specificity" is the proportion of times that a negative score reflects a true negative result; ie, the percentage of subjects who do not later display the measure's positive criteria after testing negative for drug abuse.

A tool with high sensitivity will correctly identify most patients with potential drug-abuse problems but may also incorrectly identify as high risk some patients who will not demonstrate problems with drug abuse (a false-positive result). Likewise, a tool with high specificity will correctly identify most patients who do not exhibit substance abuse but may also incorrectly identify as negative patients who do have a potential substance-abuse problem (a false-negative result). Therefore, a tool with low sensitivity will fail to identify many patients who will abuse drugs, and a tool with low specificity will fail to identify many patients who will not abuse drugs.

Box V-9

SOAPP Version 1.0:

Name:_____Date:_____

The following are some questions given to all patients at the Pain Management Center who are on or being considered for opioids for their pain. Please answer each question as honestly as possible. This information is for our records and will remain confidential. Your answers alone will not determine your treatment. Thank you.

Please answer the questions below using the following scale:

0 = Never, 1 = Seldom, 2 = Sometimes, 3 = Often, 4 = Very Often

1. How often do you feel that your pain is "out of control?" 0 1 2 3 4

2. How often do you have mood swings? 0 1 2 3 4

3. How often do you do things that you later regret? 0 1 2 3 4

4. How often has your family been supportive and encouraging? 0 1 2 3 4

5. How often have others told you that you have a bad temper? 0 1 2 3 4

6. Compared with other people, how often have you been in a car accident?
   0 1 2 3 4

7. How often do you smoke a cigarette within an hour after you wake up? 0 1 2 3 4

8. How often have you felt a need for higher doses of medication to treat your pain?
   0 1 2 3 4

9. How often do you take more medication than you are supposed to? 0 1 2 3 4

10. How often have any of your family members, including parents and grandparents, had a problem with alcohol or drugs? 0 1 2 3 4

11. How often have any of your close friends had a problem with alcohol or drugs?
    0 1 2 3 4

12. How often have others suggested that you have a drug or alcohol problem? 0 1 2 3 4

13. How often have you attended an Alcoholics Anonymous or Narcotics Anonymous meeting? 0 1 2 3 4

14. How often have you had a problem getting along with the doctors who prescribed your medicines? 0 1 2 3 4

15. How often have you taken medication other than the way that it was prescribed? 0 1 2 3 4

16. How often have you been seen by a psychiatrist or a mental health counselor? 0 1 2 3 4

17. How often have you been treated for an alcohol or drug problem? 0 1 2 3 4

18. How often have your medications been lost or stolen? 0 1 2 3 4

19. How often have others expressed concern over your use of medication? 0 1 2 3 4

20. How often have you felt a craving for medication? 0 1 2 3 4

21. How often has more than 1 doctor prescribed pain medication for you at the same time? 0 1 2 3 4

22. How often have you been asked to give a urine for substance abuse? 0 1 2 3 4

23. How often have you used illegal drugs (for example, marijuana, cocaine, etc) in the past 5 years? 0 1 2 3 4

24. How often in your lifetime have you had legal problems or been arrested? 0 1 2 3 4

Of the 24 questions contained in the SOAPP version 1.0, 16 have been identified as empirically predicting aberrant behavior 6 months after initial testing.

To score the SOAPP, ratings of the following questions are added:

2, 6, 7, 10, 11, 12, 13, 14, 15, 17, 18, 19, 20, 22, 23, 24

A score of 7 or higher is considered positive. Information on the SOAPP is available online.[23]

> **Box V:10**
>
> ## Screening Instrument for Substance Abuse Potential
>
> 1. If you drink alcohol, how many drinks do you have on a typical day?
> 2. How many drinks do you have in a typical week?
> 3. Have you used marijuana or hashish in the past year?
> 4. Have you ever smoked cigarettes?
> 5. What is your age?
>
> ### Interpretation of results from the Screening Instrument for Substance Abuse Potential
>
> Use caution when prescribing opioids for the following types of patients:
> 1. Men who consume 5 or more drinks per day or 17 or more drinks per week.
> 2. Women who consume 4 or more drinks per day or 13 or more drinks per week.
> 3. Patients who admit to marijuana or hashish use in the past year.
> 4. Patients younger than 40 years who smoke.

The meaning of a test's results can be observed in that test's negative and positive predictive values. A positive score on a test with high positive predictive power means that the problem tested for will probably be present. A negative score on a test with high negative predictive power means that the problem tested for will probably be absent. Tests that are effective in identifying patients who are at high risk for opioid abuse often produce false-positive results. Therefore, a test with a high degree of sensitivity is likely to correctly classify as high risk a patient who goes on to exhibit aberrant behaviors, but it may also classify patients as high risk who do not display problems. The current version of the SOAPP is a good example.[23] That tool's sensitivity is high; it correctly identifies about 90% of patients who will display aberrant behavior. However, about 30% of people with a high score do not display aberrant behavior.

The ORT effectively predicted the behavior of high-risk and low-risk patients but was less clear in determining the significance of the moderate-risk group.[20] Patients whose score placed them in the middle category of the ORT were as likely as not to display aberrant behavior.

In general, the wide net cast by tools that are sensitive enough to detect high-risk patients may classify many patients who do not go on to abuse drugs as being potential abusers. This may be an acceptable tradeoff until those tools can be refined. From a clinical perspective, it is better to falsely identify a person as a high-risk opioid consumer than to fail to identify a person who will harm himself or herself by abusing substances. Stigma should not be a factor in the diagnosis of having the propensity to abuse drugs, because the classification is "high-risk patient," not "substance abuser." If, as a result, the individual is at first more stringently monitored than is necessary, no harm is done. The monitoring level can be adjusted after an acceptable level of compliance has been established. But a person who may abuse drugs and is insufficiently monitored is more likely to incur harm while attempting to manage opioid intake.

Honesty in Self-Reporting

Self-reporting is always subject to inaccuracy or dishonesty from the patient who provides the information. It is logical to suspect that a person whose opioid use is out of control might fail to report his or her history of substance abuse to the person who will be providing opioids. This is particularly so for individuals intent on criminal diversion, an act that is usually well camouflaged. However, patients are often surprisingly honest when discussing substance-use disorders with healthcare professionals. The results of the ORT, which was administered in an interdisciplinary pain clinic,[20] showed that most patients responded honestly, even when asked sensitive questions about prior substance abuse. To our knowledge, data that support or refute the validity of a self-administered test about drug abuse (as opposed to an interview format) do not exist. It is probably true that a certain depth of investigation is lost when clinicians are unable to gauge, via verbal cues and facial expressions, a patient's response in person. However, such interpretations require special training that is not available in most pain-treatment settings. The widespread clinical utility of a self-administered tool renders it practical, and the accompanying savings in time and clinical resources are probably worth the tradeoff.

It is important to build trust and rapport during the assessment process to encourage and facilitate the honest sharing of information. The validity of the information provided is enhanced when:

- Confidentiality is observed.
- Patients fear no negative consequences from disclosing information.
- The information disclosed has a likelihood of subsequent verification.
- The clinician is nonjudgmental and matter-of-fact.
- The clinician treats substance-use questions as an important and routine component (like data on diet, exercise, and smoking incidence) of each patient's medical history.

Experts on substance-abuse counseling tend to declare that confrontational approaches on the subject of substance use are less effective than empathetic ones. A caring, nonjudgmental clinician who is nonetheless willing to set and implement treatment boundaries provides an indispensable component of good medical care.

Future Directions

Tools such as the ORT, the SOAPP, the PDUQ, and the SISAP, which are geared to the assessment of patients for whom opioids are prescribed, herald a new direction for researchers. Those evaluations fulfill many of the needs of opioid-treated patients. However, more testing is needed to confirm their usefulness among chronic-pain patients and to assess their validity in a variety of clinical settings. The chief quest is to discover which questions elicit answers that reliably predict who is at risk for opioid abuse. Initial testing on these newer opioid-specific tools suggest that a brief assessment may be as valid as or more so than a lengthier one. As research continues, it will likely be devoted to discovering the briefest and most accurate assessments possible. That emphasis is already apparent. The question "Has your use of alcohol or other drugs ever caused a problem for you or those close to you?" has been shown to have good validity in screening patients for prior addic-

Box V:11

Protocol for the Assessment of Patients
for the Risk of Opioid Abuse

Initial Clinic Visit:

Administer screen selected according to the clinician's expertise, time available, and clinic resources.

Brief Tests:

Opioid Risk Tool
Screener and Opioid Assessment for Patients with Pain
CAGE-Adapted to Include Drugs
Two-Item Conjoint Screen
Screening Instrument for Substance Abuse Potential

Opioid-Specific Tests:

Opioid Risk Tool
Screener and Opioid Assessment for Patients with Pain
Prescription Drug Use Questionnaire
Screening Instrument for Substance Abuse Potential

Answers to substance-related questions in briefer tests indicate the need for in-depth assessment:

Addiction Severity Index (useful for making treatment-related decisions)
Structured Clinical Interview (a thorough assessment)
Prescription Drug Use Questionnaire (particularly useful tool for opioid-treated patients)
Severity of Opiate Dependence Questionnaire (used to check for the presence and severity of opiate dependence)

Ongoing Assessment:
- Titrate medication to an analgesic dose.
- Watch for aberrant behavior.
- Document.
- Address aberrant behavior with the patient.
- Watch for the development of patterns that suggest substance abuse.
- Maintain or adjust treatment.

tion.[25] In theory, if the answer is positive, a more detailed assessment and increased monitoring are indicated if opioids are prescribed.

As previously mentioned in Chapter III, Compton and colleagues, who developed the 42-question PDUQ, discovered that 3 items on that test correctly identified addicted or nonaddicted subjects in 92% of the cases studied.[19] These items addressed the tendency to:

- Increase analgesic dose or frequency.
- Have a preferred route of drug administration.
- Consider oneself addicted.

Although the researchers concluded that it is much too early to reduce the questionnaire to these 3 questions, they lauded the clinical utility of such a reduction if it could be adequately supported by data.[19]

Ideally, tools used to assess for potential drug abuse should identify not only the individuals predisposed to abuse but also those who may abuse drugs if they are stressed past a breaking point. Pain is one of the stressful factors that, if uncontrolled, can cause drug abuse in individuals who otherwise would not be vulnerable to a substance-use disorder.

Choosing an Assessment Tool

The choice of which assessment tool to use depends on the clinician's expertise or access to specialists in the field, the time available, and other aspects of the clinical situation (Box V:11). For new patients, predictive tools can help clinicians assess potential risk before treatment begins. For a current patient, when a pattern of aberrant behavior is suspected, a diagnostic tool would be helpful. Pending further research, clinicians should assess patients by using the best available combination of questions found to be associated with the risk. The choice of which instruments or formats to use is less important than the implementation of an assessment strategy as part of routine practice. The goal is an environment in which opioids can be safely prescribed and consumed.

Ongoing Assessment

As opioid therapy progresses, clinicians must perform ongoing assessments, not only to screen for drug-related behaviors but to ensure that pain is adequately controlled and that goals for improved physical function and quality of life are met. The clinician should be especially alert to signs of stress in the patient's life. The display of any one aberrant behavior does not automatically indicate a problem with abuse or addiction. Still, such behaviors must always be:

- Documented.
- Addressed with the patient.
- Watched for the development of a pattern.

More on these subjects will follow in the chapter on monitoring patients to minimize abuse.

Conclusion

All clinicians who prescribe opioids for chronic pain should assess drug-abuse risk in their patients. The goal is not to deny pain treatment to any patient but to set and maintain a level of monitoring proportionate to the individual's risk. Patients at higher risk will require more careful monitoring and greater clinical vigilance. The clinician should remain mindful that these patients have the same rights to adequate analgesia as do low-risk or moderate-risk patients.

Each clinical practice can tailor its assessment method by taking into account the resources and expertise of the clinician. If a formal assessment is not used, the clinician must still make some effort to assess patients for the risk of drug abuse. Most importantly, patients who are at high risk should be identified before the initiation of opioid therapy and directed to appropriate treatment for the disorders that place them at high risk. The hope is that this awareness will result in better clinical outcomes and fewer instances of drug abuse.

References

1. Robinson RC, Gatchel RJ, Polatin P, Deschner M, Noe C, Gajraj N. Screening for problematic prescription opioid use. Clin J Pain. 2001 Sep;17(3):220-8.
2. Brown GS, Hermann R, Jones E, Wu J. Using self-report to improve substance abuse risk assessment in behavioral health care. Jt Comm J Qual Saf. 2004 Aug;30(8):448-54.
3. National Institute on Drug Abuse, National Institutes of Health, US Department of Health and Human Services. Research report series – prescription drugs: abuse and addiction. NIH Publication No. 01-4881. Rockville, MD. Printed 2001. Revised August 2005.
4. Sipkoff M. Pain management: health plans need to take control. Managed Care Magazine; 2003 October. MediMedia USA. Available at: http://www.managedcaremag.com/archives/0310/0310.pain.html. Accessed April 9, 2007.
5. Friedmann PD, McCullough D, Saitz R. Screening and intervention for illicit drug abuse: a national survey of primary care physicians and psychiatrists. Arch Intern Med. 2001 Jan 22;161(2):248-51.
6. Kranzler HR, Kadden RM, Babor TF, Tennen H, Rounsaville BJ. Validity of the SCID in substance abuse patients. Addiction. 1996 Jun;91(6):859-68.
7. McLellan AT, Kushner H, Metzger D, Peters R, Smith I, Grissom G, Pettinati H, Argeriou M. The fifth edition of the Addiction Severity Index. J Subst Abuse Treat. 1992;9(3):199-213.
8. Ewing JA. Detecting alcoholism. The CAGE questionnaire. JAMA. 1984 Oct 12;252(14):1905-7.
9. Brown RL, Leonard T, Saunders LA, Papasouliotis O. A two-item conjoint screen for alcohol and other drug problems. J Am Board Fam Pract. 2001 Mar-Apr;14(2):95-106.
10. Storgaard H, Nielsen SD, Gluud C. The validity of the Michigan Alcoholism Screening Test (MAST). Alcohol Alcohol 1994 Sep;29(5):493-502.

11. Davis LJ Jr, Hurt RD, Morse RM, O'Brien PC. Discriminant analysis of the Self-Administered Alcoholism Screening Test. Alcohol Clin Exp Res. 1987 Jun;11(3):269-73.
12. Saunders JB, Aasland OG, Babor TF, de la Fuente JR, Grant M. Development of the Alcohol Use Disorders Identification Test (AUDIT): WHO Collaborative Project on Early Detection of Persons with Harmful Alcohol Consumption—II. Addiction. 1993 Jun;88(6):791-804.
13. Fiellin DA, Reid MC, O'Connor PG. Screening for alcohol problems in primary care: a systematic review. Arch Intern Med. 2000 Jul 10;160(13):1977-89.
14. Brown RL, Rounds LA. Conjoint screening questionnaires for alcohol and other drug abuse: criterion validity in a primary care practice. Wis Med J. 1995;94(3):135-40.
15. Gavin DR, Ross HE, Skinner HA. Diagnostic validity of the drug abuse screening test in the assessment of DSM-III drug disorders. Br J Addict. 1989 Mar;84(3):301-7.
16. Bastiaens L, Riccardi K, Sakhrani D. The RAFFT as a screening tool for adult substance use disorders. Am J Drug Alcohol Abuse. 2002 Nov;28(4):681-91.
17. Lazowski LE, Miller FG, Boye MW, Miller GA. Efficacy of the Substance Abuse Subtle Screening Inventory-3 (SASSI-3) in identifying substance dependence disorders in clinical settings. J Pers Assess. 1998 Aug;71(1):114-28.
18. Sutherland G, Edwards G, Taylor C, Phillips G, Gossop M, Brady R. The measurement of opiate dependence. Br J Addict. 1986 Aug;81(4):485-94.
19. Compton P, Darakjian J, Miotto K. Screening for addiction in patients with chronic pain and "problematic" substance use: evaluation of a pilot assessment tool. J Pain Symptom Manage. 1998 Dec;16(6):355-63.
20. Webster LR, Webster RM. Predicting aberrant behaviors in opioid-treated patients: preliminary validation of the Opioid Risk Tool. Pain Med. 2005 Nov-Dec;6(6):432-42.
21. Butler SF, Budman SH, Fernandez K, Jamison RN. Validation of a screener and opioid assessment measure for patients with chronic pain. Pain. 2004 Nov;112(1-2):65-75.
22. Akbik H, Butler SF, Budman SH, Fernandez K, Katz NP, Jamison RN. Validation and clinical application of the Screener and Opioid Assessment for Patients with Pain (SOAPP). J Pain Symptom Manage. 2006 Sep;32(3):287-93.
23. SOAPP frequently asked questions. Pain EDU.org. Available at: http://www.painedu.org/soap-development.asp. Accessed April 9, 2007.
24. Coambs RB, Jarry JL. The SISAP: a new screening instrument for identifying potential opioid abusers in the management of chronic nonmalignant pain in general medical practice. Pain Res Manage. 1996;1:15-162.
25. Fine PG, Portenoy RK. A Clinical Guide to Opioid Analgesia. Minneapolis, MN: McGraw-Hill; 2004.

CHAPTER VI

MONITORING PATIENTS TO MINIMIZE OPIOID ABUSE

Consider each opioid patient to represent a clinical
investigation with an 'N' of one.
-Lawrence M. Probes, MD, psychiatrist specializing in the treatment of chronic pain[1]

Successful opioid therapy for chronic pain consists of several important steps. Clinicians should familiarize themselves with the prevalence and mechanisms of addiction, the behaviors that signal problems with managing opioids, the risk factors for substance abuse, and the instruments used to assess the individual's personal risk for substance abuse. All this enables the clinician to prescribe the most effective treatment. What happens next determines whether the entire treatment plan fails or succeeds: Each patient must be monitored for his or her response to opioid treatment. The commitment to maintaining vigilance begins on the initial clinic visit and continues for as long as therapy lasts.

Some degree of monitoring should take place during each and every visit. The focus should be on the patient's degree of pain relief, physical function, quality of life, and any drug-related aberrant behaviors that have arisen. Patients at higher risk for opioid abuse or addiction require stringent clinical vigilance if opioids are to be prescribed appropriately.

In this chapter, the items that should be documented in the patient's chart are specified and the advantages and limitations of treatment contracts and urine drug screenings are reviewed. Clinicians will get a sense of which monitoring tools are most appropriate for different risk levels.

Getting the Patient Started

Monitoring a patient who is treated with long-term opioid therapy means checking for the effectiveness of pain treatment and signs of abuse or addiction involving opioids. A primary maxim is to prevent harm, which can stem from several sources, including uncontrolled drug use, unmanageable adverse effects, or an increase in pain.

The Initial Visit

Because good monitoring begins when the patient first enters the medical establishment, clinicians should follow a template to reduce the chances of missing important data. Several good guides are available, and clinicians can modify and personalize them according to their own needs. After a template has been selected, it should be used consistently. An example is the guide to opioid prescribing outlined by the American Academy of Pain Medicine (AAPM) and the American Pain Society (APS).[2] The discussion that follows uses that guide's 5 recommended steps as a framework and then expands them.

1) Conduct a thorough patient evaluation. Begin with a patient interview followed by a complete physical examination. The chart should contain the patient's:

- Chief complaint.
- Medical history.
- Pain history.
- Diagnostic findings.
- Results and analyses of laboratory tests and screenings.
- All drugs and interventions tried.
- Substance-abuse history.
- Results of substance-abuse assessment.
- Comorbid conditions, including any mood or sleep disorders.
- Work history.

When the patient is reassessed at each visit, the clinician should remain alert for the effect of substance use and pain on the patient's work, family relationships, social activities, and all other facets of life.

2) *Craft an individualized treatment plan.* After having analyzed the findings from step 1, the clinician should partner with the patient to develop a treatment plan that is:

- Designed specifically for the patient.
- Tailored to the patient's current complaint.
- Based on realistic treatment goals that have been discussed with the patient.
- Mindful of the outcome of all prior treatment modalities.
- Clear about the potential risks and benefits of opioid therapy.
- Flexible enough to incorporate adjustments when needed.

This step may include a written opioid treatment agreement that outlines expectations and specifies the consequences of noncompliance.

3) *Access consultation as needed.* The clinician should consider consulting with experts in other fields to facilitate needed concurrent treatment. Such experts could include:

- Pain specialists.
- Psychologists.
- Psychiatrists.
- Physical therapists.
- Addiction specialists.
- Alternative therapists.
- Twelve-step groups or other support groups.

4) *Introduce periodic review of treatment efficacy.* Patients who receive long-term opioid therapy must be reassessed frequently. Each clinic visit is an opportunity to note the following:

- Degree of pain relief.
- Physical function (change from baseline).
- Psychosocial function.

- Quality of life (meaningful to patient).
- Adverse effects and how they are being managed.
- Progress toward treatment goals.
- Indications of medication misuse and how any problem is being addressed.

5) Document, document, document. The importance of complete written records cannot be overemphasized. Incomplete or inaccurate documentation can compromise the patient's care. Now more than ever (and especially in the event of any legal questions), the treatment choices and the reasons those therapies were selected must be recorded. It is also advisable in some instances to state the reasons nonopioid treatment was not pursued. The documentation must detail:

- The outcome of all items listed in step 4 (the periodic review).
- The reason for opioid treatment.
- Adjustments to the treatment plan, including changes in dosage.
- Any further interventions, surgeries, tests, etc.
- Reports from consultants.
- The content of any directives or counseling given to the patient.

Setting Treatment Goals

A feasible treatment plan must include goals that are personal to the patient. Those goals must also be realistic. Although opioids are still the best treatment available for the relief of moderate-to-severe pain, they are more effective against some types of pain than against other types, and they do not completely eliminate most pain. Opioids are not a cure for chronic pain; they are a useful tool in its treatment. Part of effectively prescribing opioids includes managing unrealistic patient expectations. Counseling patients about setting achievable treatment goals is like walking a tightrope. It is unwise to dampen a patient's hopes by declaring, "You will simply have to learn to live with this pain." Such statements may be clinically inaccurate. No clinician can read the future, and the mind-body connection in pain control has been well established. Hope is a powerful healer and can be a tremendous aid in helping patients to meet their goals. Although most chronic pain is unlikely to be completely eliminated, opioids do confer significant benefits for many patients. In 1 survey of 388 opioid-treated chronic-pain patients, 78% described the degree of pain relief they achieved as meaningful.[3] Ample evidence supports the wisdom of helping patients keep hope alive.

The success of opioid therapy depends on the specific priorities of the patient. A patient with advanced cancer may desire only noninvasive palliative care. For a patient with chronic nonmalignant pain, the benefits of opioids should be weighed against their disadvantages. Determining the patient's priorities in treatment is essential. What is most important to the patient? That he or she:

- Feels less pain?
- Avoids feeling groggy or sedated?
- Stays within certain cost or insurance limits?
- Avoids appearing dependent on drugs?

Often, patient priorities can be measured in terms of physical function. What does the patient wish to accomplish that the pain is now making impossible? Examples could include regaining the ability to:

• Return to work.
• Care for children and handle household responsibilities.
• Drive.
• Exercise.
• Leave bed for a holiday celebration with relatives.
• Attend a special event outside the home.
• Return to engaging in a competitive sport.
• Walk to the corner grocer.

The goals of individual patients can cover a wide range of possibilities. For example:

> A 74-year-old woman has severe degeneration of the spine. Her compressed vertebrae have been treated with vertebral plasties, but her function continues to be limited because of the pain in her back that occurs during ambulation. She would be satisfied if she could walk for 20 minutes a day without excruciating pain.

Helping patients to articulate their own needs and priorities helps them own the treatment process and strengthens their commitment to following medical direction. The usual first step to setting reasonable treatment goals is to delineate all expectations associated with opioid therapy in a written treatment agreement.

Setting Boundaries: The Opioid Treatment Agreement

It is critical to keep complete written patient records that detail the rationale and progress of long-term opioid therapy. The treatment agreement initiates this practice and sets the tone for the patient-clinician relationship. This immediate establishment of structure can improve the therapeutic relationship as long as it is accompanied by open dialogue. An opioid treatment agreement should:

• Detail the goals of therapy.
• Establish the responsibilities of the clinician and the patient.
• Provide information about the adverse effects and risks of treatment.
• Set boundaries for compliance.
• Establish consequences for failure to follow medical direction.
• Encourage the patient to take responsibility for his or her treatment.

The agreement should be signed by the patient and the provider and possibly also by other healthcare professionals involved in the patient's care. At every step, the patient should be held accountable for adherence to the agreement; this increases the likelihood of compliance.

Not everyone agrees on what should be included in an agreement like that described above. However, most experts now consider such a document advantageous because it initiates opioid therapy in an atmosphere of mutual trust and full disclosure. Some experts recommend having signed agreements for high-risk patients only. But in general and according to the currently accepted policy, all pain patients should sign a treatment agreement at the beginning of long-term opioid therapy. This is only a recommendation, however, and not a decree. A clinician's free agency and discretion in treating individual patients should not be compromised by guidelines that could be perceived as universally expected. That said, a treatment agreement offers significant advantages (and some cautions) for both patient and clinician.

Advantages and Limitations of Treatment Agreements

Because written documentation is more important than ever for legal purposes, having a signed record that a patient has provided informed consent for treatment is an advantage. If the medical record is ever reviewed, the examiners can quickly ascertain which information was disseminated and which treatment plan was agreed to by the patient and the provider.

Having this type of signed document also facilitates what otherwise could be a difficult discussion between patient and clinician by introducing the topic of noncompliance early and in a nonthreatening way. Providing the agreement in a standard form may prevent certain patients from feeling singled out for scrutiny. The signed agreement confers other benefits. The responsibilities of both patient and provider are clearly defined. Treatment boundaries are set, and consequences for aberrant behavior are outlined. Patients are encouraged to take responsibility for key aspects of their pain management program.

For the high-risk patient, the advantages of having a signed agreement are even greater. The establishment of unambiguous treatment goals and clear consequences for noncompliance facilitates early intervention if a patient does indeed exhibit a substance-abuse problem. The framework facilitates rapid modifications when aberrant behaviors occur.

Certain limitations of the treatment agreement do exist, however. The chief danger for a clinician is exposure to legal liability if he or she fails or is perceived to have failed to enforce the letter of the agreement. Agreements should be carefully worded, and clinicians must be prepared to enforce them. These documents should be termed "agreements" rather than "contracts," because the latter term implies a stronger legal relationship and suggests a greater obligation. Another potential liability is that such documents may cause complacency in the clinician. To obtain a signed agreement is only the beginning of good monitoring practice; ongoing clinical vigilance should not be sacrificed. Some patients may feel stigmatized or humiliated by being asked to sign such an agreement, particularly if they harbor negative feelings about long-term opioid therapy. To combat that attitude, the clinician should present the document as a matter of clinical course – as a medical issue and not a moral judgment.

Questions remain regarding how effective these agreements are in ensuring patient compliance. No strong evidence as yet supports the practice as a motivating force for adherence. The tide of support for agreements comes primarily from pain experts in the field who testify to their clinical efficacy. To craft an agreement that is useful without being too rigid, some thought should be given to the specific language used. What is omitted from the document may be as important as what is included.

What Should a Treatment Agreement Contain?

An example of an agreement and an informed consent can be seen in Box VI:1. It is also acceptable to combine the 2 documents into 1. Attorney Jennifer Bolen, who specializes in the legal and regulatory compliance issues of pain medicine, advises clinicians to craft documents using the same terminology as the controlled-substance rules of their home state.[4] Content may vary but should contain some variation of the following fundamentals:

- The goals of opioid treatment.
- The specification of 1 physician and 1 pharmacy to prescribe and dispense the patient's opioids.
- The risks and potential adverse effects of opioid treatment, including an acknowledgement that patients with a history of substance abuse may be at risk for the recurrence of abuse.
- A mention of available alternatives to treat pain.
- Correct definitions of addiction, tolerance, and physical dependence.
- A request for patient disclosure of his or her substance-abuse history and current medications.
- An explanation regarding a patient's responsibility to safeguard medications.
- A description of the need at each medical visit for the complete and honest self-report of pain relief, adverse effects of treatment, and function.
- A description of the behaviors that constitute noncompliance, such as unauthorized escalation of dosages, the selling or lending of medications, or the mixing of medications with illegal street drugs or unauthorized prescriptions.
- The consequences of noncompliance.
- The signature of the provider and the patient. A specialist should consider securing the signature and cooperation of the patient's primary care physician as well.

The best agreements also provide for:
- Regular appointments to review the treatment plan.
- Regular prescription refills during normal office hours.
- Patient consent for random urine drug testing or medication counts.
- Patient waiver of privacy to contact other providers to discuss patient care.
- The patient's promise to disclose whether he or she visits a hospital emergency department and receives controlled substances.
- The option of sharing information with certain family members as needed.
- A pledge from substance abusers to enter and maintain a recovery program.

A critical component of the opioid treatment agreement is the mandate that only 1 provider control all access to opioids. The patient may choose the pharmacy but cannot change pharmacies after that initial selection has been made. The description of the risks of opioid therapy should include some mention of the possibility that opioid treatment can result in dependence, tolerance, or addiction. Consequences for breaking the agreement should be clearly listed. Each clinician must set parameters that feel comfortable and enforceable. Because of the prevalence of noncompliance in clinical practice, dismissing a patient at the first offense is probably too harsh. A first offense could require counseling, for instance, and a second offense or the appearance of more serious behaviors could trigger intensified monitoring, such as more frequent

Box VI:1   **Example of Agreement for Long-term Opioid Use:[21]**

The purpose of this agreement is to protect your access to controlled substances and to protect our ability to prescribe for you. The long-term use of such substances as opioids (narcotic analgesics), benzodiazepine tranquilizers, and barbiturate sedatives is controversial because of uncertainty regarding the extent to which they provide long-term benefit. In people with a prior addiction, there is also the risk of the development of an addictive disorder or a recurrence of drug abuse. The extent of that risk is uncertain.

Because these drugs have potential for abuse or diversion, strict accountability is necessary when use is prolonged. For this reason, the following policies are agreed to by you (the patient) as a condition of the willingness of the physician whose signature appears below to consider the initial and/or continued prescription of controlled substances to treat your chronic pain.

1. Unless specific authorization is obtained for an exception, all controlled substances must come ONLY from the physicians or nurse practitioners at Lifetree Pain Clinic. You will not attempt to get pain medication from any other healthcare provider without telling him or her that you are taking pain medication prescribed by this clinic. You understand that failing to provide that information to a prescriber is against the law. If your primary care physician is willing to prescribe your medications, this clinic will have to approve the arrangements to ensure that there is no duplication. <u>You will discontinue all previously used pain medications unless you are told to continue them.</u> All controlled substances must be obtained at the same pharmacy, if possible. If the need to change pharmacies arises, our office must be informed. The pharmacy that you have selected is:

_____

Phone: _____

2. You are expected to inform our office of any new medications or medical conditions and of any adverse effects you experience from any of the medications that you take.
3. To maintain accountability, the prescribing physician has permission to discuss all diagnostic and treatment details with dispensing pharmacists or other professionals who provide your healthcare information. You agree to waive any applicable privilege or right of privacy or confidentiality with respect to the prescribing of your pain medication, and you authorize the clinic and your pharmacy to cooperate fully with any city, state, or federal law enforcement agency, including the state Department of Professional and Occupational Licensing, in the investigation of any possible misuse, sale, or other diversion of your pain medication. You authorize the clinic to provide a copy of this agreement to your pharmacy.
4. You may not share, sell, or otherwise permit others to have access to these medications.
5. Do not stop taking these drugs abruptly, because abstinence syndrome will likely develop.
6. Unannounced urine or serum toxicology screenings may be requested, and your cooperation is required. The presence of an unauthorized substance may prompt an adjustment in your treatment and monitoring.
7. Prescriptions and bottles of these medications may be sought by individuals with chemical dependency and should be closely safeguarded. It is expected that you will take

the highest possible degree of care with your medications and prescriptions. They should not be left where others might see or otherwise have access to them.

8. Original containers of medications may be required for you to bring to office visits.

9. Because these drugs may be hazardous or lethal to people (especially children) who are not tolerant of their effects, you must keep the drugs away from those people.

10. Medications may not be replaced if they are lost, get wet, are destroyed, are left on an airplane, etc. Such events may cause your treatment to be reassessed, and an alternative therapy may be prescribed.

11. Refills will be given only at the discretion of the provider. The preparation of all refills requires advance notice of three (3) business days. Early refills will not be given unless the provider feels that there is justification to do so.

12. Prescription renewals are contingent upon your keeping scheduled appointments. All prescriptions will be given on weekdays, Monday through Friday, from 9:00 AM to 4:00 PM. Prescriptions will NOT be given at any other time unless extreme extraordinary circumstances apply.

13. If the responsible legal authorities have questions concerning your treatment (eg, whether you were obtaining medications at several pharmacies) all confidentiality is waived, and those authorities may be given full access to our records of controlled-substance administration (as stated in item #3).

14. It is understood that failure to adhere to these policies may result in the cessation of therapy with controlled-substance prescribing by this physician or referral for further specialty assessment.

15. It should be understood that any medical treatment is initially a trial and that continued prescribing is contingent upon evidence of benefit.

16. The risks and potential benefits of these therapies are explained elsewhere. You must acknowledge that you have received that explanation.

17. You affirm that you have full right and power to sign and be bound by this agreement and that you have read, understood, and accepted its terms.

18. You are advised not to drive while you are being treated with any medication we prescribe without having had an appropriate driver's test that indicates that it is safe for you to drive.

If any of the above conditions is violated, the provider may choose to wean you off opioid medication, and your painful condition will be managed without the use of opioids. Further opioids may not be prescribed for any chronic painful condition that may develop. Violations of the above-stated terms might also result in your being discharged from the clinic with appropriate written notice and warning and without receiving weaning medications or treatment from Lifetree Pain Clinic.

_____
Physician signature

_____
Patient signature

_____
Date

_____
Patient name (printed)

Example of Informed Consent for Long-Term Opioid Therapy

The Providers at Lifetree Pain Clinic are prescribing opioid medicine, sometimes called narcotic analgesics, to me for a diagnosis of:

_____

This decision was made because my condition is serious or other treatments have not helped my pain.

I am aware that the use of such medicine has certain risks that include but are not limited to sleepiness or drowsiness, constipation, nausea, itching, vomiting, dizziness, allergic reaction, slowing of the breathing rate, slowing of reflexes or reaction time, and (possibly) inadequate pain relief.

I am aware of the possible risks and benefits of other types of treatments that do not involve the use of opioids. The other treatments discussed included:

_____

I will tell my doctor about all other medicines and treatments that I am receiving.

I will not be involved in any activity that may be dangerous to me or someone else if I feel drowsy or am not thinking clearly. Such activities include but are not limited to using heavy equipment or driving a motor vehicle, working at a height while unprotected, or being responsible for another individual who is unable to care for himself or herself. I am aware that even if I do not notice it, my reflexes and reaction time might still be slowed. I have been advised not to drive while receiving treatment with any medication prescribed without having passed an appropriate driver's test indicating that it is safe to drive.

I am aware that addiction is defined as the use of a medication even if it causes harm, having cravings for a drug, feeling the need to use a drug, and having a decreased quality of life. I am aware that there is a chance of becoming addicted to my pain medicine, but that the risk is low. I am aware that the development of addiction is much more common in a person who has a family or personal history of addiction. I agree to tell my doctor my complete and honest personal drug history and that of my family to the best of my knowledge.

I understand that physical dependence is a normal and expected result of using these medicines for a long time. I understand that physical dependence is not the same as addiction. I am aware that physical dependence means that if my pain medicine use is markedly decreased, stopped, or reversed by some of the agents mentioned above, I will experience a withdrawal syndrome. This means that I may have any or all of the following signs and symptoms: a runny nose, yawning, large pupils, goose bumps, abdominal pain and cramping, diarrhea, irritability, aches throughout my body, and a flu-like feeling. I am aware that opioid withdrawal is uncomfortable but not life-threatening.

I am aware that tolerance to analgesia means that I may require more medicine to obtain the same amount of pain relief. I am aware that tolerance to analgesia does not seem to be a major problem for most patients with chronic pain; however, such tolerance has been noted, and I may experience it. If tolerance occurs, increasing doses may not always help and may cause unacceptable adverse effects. Tolerance or failure to respond well to opioid treatment may cause my doctor to choose another form of treatment.

(Men ONLY) I am aware that long-term opioid use has been associated with a low testosterone level in men. This may affect my mood, stamina, sexual desire, and physical and sexual performance. I understand that my doctor may check my blood to see if my testosterone level is normal.

(Women ONLY) If I plan to become pregnant or believe that I have become pregnant while taking this pain medicine, I will immediately call my obstetrician and this office to inform them. I am aware that, should I carry a baby to term while I am taking these medicines, the baby will be physically dependent upon opioids. I am aware that the use of opioids is not usually associated with the risk of birth defects. However, birth defects can occur whether or not a mother is treated with medication, and there is always the possibility that my child will be born with a birth defect if I take an opioid while I am pregnant.

I have read this form or have had it read to me. I understand all of it. I have had an opportunity to have all of my questions regarding this treatment answered to my satisfaction. By signing this form voluntarily, I give my consent for the treatment of my pain with opioid pain-management medicines.

_____

Physician signature

_____

Patient signature

_____

Date

_____

Patient name (printed)

Box VI:2

The Pain Assessment and Documentation Tool

PROGRESS NOTE
Pain Assessment and Documentation Tool (PADT™)

Patient Stamp Here

Patient Name: _____ Record #: _____

Assessment Date: _____

Current Analgesic Regimen

Drug name	Strength (eg, mg)	Frequency	Maximum Total Daily Dose
_____	_____	_____	_____
_____	_____	_____	_____
_____	_____	_____	_____

The PADT is a clinician-directed interview; that is, the clinician asks the questions, and the clinician records the responses. The Analgesia, Activities of Daily Living, and Adverse Events sections may be completed by the physician, nurse practitioner, physician assistant, or nurse. The Potential Aberrant Drug-Related Behavior and Assessment sections must be completed by the __physician__. Ask the patient the questions below, except as noted.

Analgesia

If zero indicates "no pain" and ten indicates "pain as bad as it can be," on a scale of 0 to 10, what is your level of pain for the following questions?

1. What was your pain level on average during the past week? (Please circle the appropriate number)

No Pain 0 1 2 3 4 5 6 7 8 9 10 **Pain as bad as it can be**

2. What was your pain level at its worst during the past week?

No Pain 0 1 2 3 4 5 6 7 8 9 10 **Pain as bad as it can be**

3. What percentage of your pain has been relieved during the past week? (Write in a percentage between 0% and 100%.) _____

4. Is the amount of pain relief you are now obtaining from your current pain reliever(s) enough to make a real difference in your life?
❑ Yes   ❑ No

5. Query to clinician: Is the patient's pain relief clinically significant?
❑ Yes   ❑ No   ❑ Unsure

Activities of Daily Living

Please indicate whether the patient's functioning with the current pain reliever(s) is Better, the Same, or Worse since the patient's last assessment with the PADT.* (Please check the box for Better, Same, or Worse for each item below.)

	Better	Same	Worse
1. Physical functioning	❑	❑	❑
2. Family relationships	❑	❑	❑
3. Social relationships	❑	❑	❑
4. Mood	❑	❑	❑
5. Sleep patterns	❑	❑	❑
6. Overall functioning	❑	❑	❑

* If the patient is receiving his or her first PADT assessment, the clinician should compare the patient's functional status with other reports from the last office visit.

(Continued on reverse side)

Box VI:2

The Pain Assessment and Documentation Tool

PROGRESS NOTE
Pain Assessment and Documentation Tool (PADT™)

Adverse Events

1. Is patient experiencing any side effects from current pain reliever(s)? ❑ Yes ❑ No

Ask patient about potential side effects:

	None	Mild	Moderate	Severe
a. Nausea	❑	❑	❑	❑
b. Vomiting	❑	❑	❑	❑
c. Constipation	❑	❑	❑	❑
d. Itching	❑	❑	❑	❑
e. Mental cloudiness	❑	❑	❑	❑
f. Sweating	❑	❑	❑	❑
g. Fatigue	❑	❑	❑	❑
h. Drowsiness	❑	❑	❑	❑
i. Other _____	❑	❑	❑	
j. Other _____	❑	❑	❑	

2. Patient's overall severity of side effects?
❑ None   ❑ Mild   ❑ Moderate   ❑ Severe

Potential Aberrant Drug-Related Behavior
This section must be completed by the <u>physician</u>.

Please **check** *any of the following items that you discovered during your interactions with the patient.* Please note that some of these are directly observable (eg, appears intoxicated), while others may require more active listening and/or probing. Use the "Assessment" section below to note additional details.

❑ Purposeful over-sedation
❑ Negative mood change
❑ Appears intoxicated
❑ Increasingly unkempt or impaired
❑ Involvement in car or other accident
❑ Requests frequent early renewals
❑ Increased dose without authorization
❑ Reports lost or stolen prescriptions
❑ Attempts to obtain prescriptions from other doctors
❑ Changes route of administration
❑ Uses pain medication in response to situational stressor
❑ Insists on certain medications by name
❑ Contact with street drug culture
❑ Abusing alcohol or illicit drugs
❑ Hoarding (ie, stockpiling) of medication
❑ Arrested by police
❑ Victim of abuse
Other: _____
_____
_____

Assessment: (This section must be completed by the <u>physician</u>.)
Is your overall impression that this patient is benefiting (eg, benefits, such as pain relief, outweigh side effects) from opioid therapy?   ❑ Yes   ❑ No   ❑ Unsure

Comments: _____
_____

Specific Analgesic Plan:
❑ Continue present regimen   Comments: _____
❑ Adjust dose of present analgesic   _____
❑ Switch analgesics   _____
❑ Add/Adjust concomitant therapy   _____
❑ Discontinue/taper off opioid therapy   _____

Date: _____   Physician's signature: _____

Provided as a service to the medical community by Janssen Pharmaceutica Products, L.P.   JANSSEN ▣   PHARMACEUTICA PRODUCTS, L.P.

office visits or random drug screening. Time is an important factor. If, for example, a first offense occurs in January and a second offense occurs 1 year later, this is not as problematic as if the behaviors occurred 2 weeks apart. The contract could specify that continuing offenses will result in escalating penalties up to and including termination. The contract could also contain "deal breakers" (eg, illegal activities such as forgery or the selling of prescriptions) that call for the immediate cessation of opioid therapy.

Most experts agree that the language in an agreement should allow the clinician "wiggle room" in discharging patients so that each case of noncompliance is decided on an individual basis. For example, in describing behaviors that are the basis for dismissal from care, most experts recommend the use of the phrase "may dismiss" instead of "will dismiss" to avoid compromising independent clinical judgment. However, such a clause could also cause legal trouble for a clinician if it does not clearly list the conditions under which a patient will definitely be terminated. Because the implications of and for dismissal have not been established, clinicians must choose language based on their best judgment. In general, though, ultimatums should be avoided because they limit the choices of the clinician.

It is also worthwhile to consider adding to the written agreement a section giving the treating clinician permission to seek and exchange information on patient care with former providers, current mental-healthcare or addiction-treatment providers, and members of the patient's family. Specific laws protect the disclosure of patient information on mental health and substance abuse. A signed agreement can eliminate barriers to obtaining necessary information.

Two other issues to consider are whether patients treated with long-term opioid therapy should drive and whether pregnant patients should take an opioid. Driving is generally considered safe for patients who receive long-term opioids after tolerance to the sedative effects of those agents has been achieved. Patients should be advised not to drive after initial dosing with an opioid or after the dosage has been increased. The decision of whether to drive belongs to the patient alone, but such patients must understand that they should never drive under the influence of alcohol or illicit drugs, change their own medication regimen, or drive when they are feeling sedated.[5] If an employer requires proof that the patient can drive safely, the patient should take an appropriate driver's test and furnish the results to the employer.

The agreement should require the patient to notify the prescriber if pregnancy occurs or is anticipated. Medical opioid use does not appear to cause birth defects in the absence of drug abuse, but the evidence is not conclusive.

There is no universal style for writing an opioid treatment agreement. Fishman and colleagues distinguished between language that is cooperative as opposed to paternalistic.[6] The cooperative style explains why the agreement is necessary and emphasizes the patient's partnership role. This approach provides a rationale for every policy presented. The paternalistic style, which is more authoritarian, emphasizes clear guidelines and consequences for rule breaking. The clinician is free to choose language that best fits with his or her own treatment philosophy. The healthcare provider should keep a copy of the agreement in the patient's medical file and provide a copy for the patient. With a treatment agreement in hand it is much easier to accomplish the ongoing monitoring that comprises the bulk of long-term opioid treatment.

Guidelines for Monitoring Patient Progress

Most patients who begin opioid therapy for pain do so on a trial basis, and 6 weeks of treatment is a common duration for a test period. It is always vital to watch and document the patient's response to opioid therapy, but it is particularly so during this time. If the trial is deemed successful and opioid therapy is continued, regular assessments should continue for as long as the therapy is used.

The standards by which to judge the success or failure of opioid therapy are:

• Whether a patient's overall functioning and quality of life have been improved by treatment.
• Whether adverse effects and aberrant behaviors have been controlled.

Minimizing the risk of abuse and addiction relates directly to the optimal delivery of good pain management. This relationship is clear when we consider that opioid misuse impairs physical function and quality of life. Pain relief is an unlikely outcome of opioid therapy in patients who abuse their medications.

Ongoing Monitoring: The Four A's

Treatment outcomes are the standard by which to judge any medical therapy. For pain patients, a good question to keep in mind is whether the consumption of opioids appears to be improving function or causing harm. A tool such as the "Four A's" (analgesia [pain relief], activities of daily living [psychosocial functioning], adverse events [side effects of treatment], and aberrant drug taking [addiction-related outcomes]) is helpful in this regard because it can be used to evaluate the precise outcomes of greatest clinical interest when prescribing opioids for pain.[7] Every clinic visit should trigger an entry in the patient's chart for each of the 4 topics. The Pain Assessment and Documentation Tool (PADT), which is an expanded version of the Four A's and is featured in Box VI:2, provides a more in-depth means of documenting progress.[8] Tools such as the Four A's and the PADT provide a structure for noting the patient's response to treatment, any changes in therapy, and any counseling that takes place.

Analgesia

Steven Passik, PhD, who helped to develop the Four A's and the PADT, recommends that the following 4 questions pertaining to analgesia be asked of patients during each visit. The patient is asked to respond to the first 2 questions by means of a 10-point scale in which zero represents "no pain" and 10 represents "the worst pain imaginable."

• What was your pain level on average during the past week?
• What was your pain level at its worst during the past week?
• When you compare the effectiveness of your current treatment with that of your previous treatment with other pain medications, what percentage of your pain has been relieved?
• Is your current level of pain relief sufficient to make a real difference in your life?

The answers to those questions will help the clinician to determine whether the patient is responding to the treatment as hoped and whether adjustments are necessary.

Activity

Some experts argue that the goal of opioid therapy should be pain relief alone, regardless of the impact of treatment on physical function. However, function is the only objective measure of improvement, and if a patient's physical functioning improves, pain control has likely been successful. Opioids consumed long term must be incorporated into the patient's lifestyle. Therefore, it is appropriate to measure and document examples of patient activity, including:

- Sleep.
- Relationships with others.
- Mood.
- Work.
- Home responsibilities.
- Recreation.
- Family and social life.

Patients should answer whether those factors have improved, remained the same, or worsened since their last visit and also since their first assessment. After the maximum improvement has been achieved, the goal is to maintain the improvement over baseline.

Measures of function also can help determine whether a patient suffers from a true substance-use disorder. Because pain often decreases function, good analgesia that results from opioid therapy should increase activity in a patient after tolerance to the initial sedating effect of the drug has been achieved. If opioid use is restricting a patient's activity level rather than improving it, that patient may be misusing opioids to address issues other than pain control. The American Chronic Pain Association suggests that the following behaviors may signal trouble with the current opioid regimen:

- Sleeping too much or confusing night and day.
- A decrease in appetite.
- An inability to concentrate or a short attention span.
- Mood swings (especially irritability).
- Lack of involvement with others.
- Difficulty functioning caused by the effects of the drug.
- Use of drugs to regress rather than facilitate involvement in life.
- Lack of attention to appearance and hygiene.[9]

If the patient is able to fulfill responsibilities centered on work, home, social life, and family while taking pain medication, it is less likely that an abuse problem is present. It can even be said that good pain management should help promote the happiness of the patient. This is an achievable goal, even in the presence of pain that is not completely controlled. Adjustments in the treatment regimen may be needed if a medication diminishes (instead of improves) a patient's ability to enjoy life.

Adverse Events

Most patients treated with an opioid experience some adverse effects of treatment. Constipation is the most commonly reported troublesome event. The adverse effects experienced and their degree of impact, all of which are influenced by the patient's age and the opioid dosage, vary widely among patients.

To continue using the Passik approach, patients should answer the following questions:

- Are you able to tolerate your current pain relievers? (yes or no)
- Are you experiencing any adverse effects from your current pain relievers? (yes or no)
- Would you rate the severity of constipation that you are experiencing as none, mild, moderate, or severe?

The clinician then evaluates whether the treatment-related effects can be tolerated by that particular patient. Medications can be prescribed to relieve constipation. Some adverse effects take time to resolve. Tolerance to sedation usually develops quickly. A review of the pertinent literature revealed that stable doses of opioids do not appear to impair driving skills in opioid-tolerant patients.[5] Most patients are able to begin performing tasks of daily living soon after the initiation of opioid therapy.

Aberrant Behavior

The uncontrolled use of medication by the patient reduces the likelihood of achieving good pain management. Any behaviors that arise must be documented, addressed with the patient, and assessed for their potential impact on the success of therapy. The following guidelines may be useful for the ongoing monitoring of aberrant behavior in pain patients.

- Use open-ended questions that are difficult to answer evasively or that cannot be answered with a simple "yes" or "no."
- Probe and be persistent; rephrase questions.
- Don't assume anything.
- Confront discrepancies in a nonjudgmental manner.
- Express empathy.
- Let the patient know that you are there to help.
- Observe the patient's behavior for indications of denial or false information, such as avoidance of eye contact, long pauses before answering, fidgeting, or hostile gestures.
- Corroborate the patient's statements using other sources such as friends, family members, the results of physical examinations and laboratory testing, observation, and clues from the patient's medical history.

When aberrant behaviors are confirmed or strongly suspected, monitoring measures must be intensified. To do this, it is necessary to match the degree of monitoring to the level of risk for substance abuse.

Matching Monitoring to the Level of Risk

The outcome of assessment as described in Chapter V will help the clinician set the patient's level of monitoring. Whatever the patient's risk level, a variety of strategies can help ensure compliance with medical direction and prevent substance abuse. Some monitoring techniques are standard and appropriate for every patient. Others, such as the third-party administration of medication, are stricter methods that should be used in patients whose substance-abuse assessment indicates that they are either at high risk for drug abuse or have a

Box VI:3	Match Monitoring to the Patient's Risk of Drug Abuse.	
Low Risk (Routine) for Drug Abuse	**Moderate Risk for Drug Abuse**	**High Risk for Drug Abuse**
Pain assessment Substance-abuse assessment Informed consent Signed treatment agreement Regular follow-up visits, prescriptions Initial prescription database check Medical reports Initial urine drug screening No consultation required Medication type, unrestricted Document Four A's Document patient-provider interactions	Biweekly visits Biweekly prescriptions Regular prescription database check Third-party verification Random urine drug screening Consider comorbid disease Consider psychiatric/ addiction/pain evaluation Consider medication counts Consider limiting rapid-onset analgesics	Weekly visits Weekly prescriptions (on attendance) Quarterly prescription database check Third-party administration Urine drug screening, scheduled and random Consider blood screenings Psychiatric/addiction evaluation required Consider pain specialist evaluation Limit rapid-onset analgesics Consider limiting short-acting agents

confirmed problem in managing drug use (See Box VI:3). It is advisable to apply a minimum level of monitoring to all patients and then to intensify monitoring as the risk level rises. This individualizing of the monitoring process is in keeping with the universal precautions for pain practice advanced by Douglas Gourlay, MD; Howard Heit, MD; and Abdulaziz Almahrezi, MD.[10] Their minimum recommendations for all patients include:

- The diagnosis of any identifiable pain causes and comorbid conditions.
- Initial and ongoing assessment of substance use and mental health status.
- Initial and ongoing pain assessment.
- Informed consent of opioid benefits and risks.
- An opioid treatment agreement.
- A trial of appropriate medications.
- Regular assessment of the Four A's.
- Thorough documentation.

Further recommendations for low-risk, moderate-risk, and high-risk patients follow.

Low-risk patients should be monitored at a level that could be described as routine. This does not mean these individuals are not monitored with vigilance and care, only that no extraordinary measures are required.

- Explain the standard treatment agreement; both provider and patient should sign it.
- Schedule regular follow-up visits (monthly at first).
- Set the frequency of medication refills (monthly for the first 6 months).
- Perform initial urine (or other) drug screening.
- Communicate with pharmacies or obtain initial reports from prescription-monitoring programs (where available) and prior medical providers.
- Document every patient and clinician interaction.
- Continually review the Four A's during return visits.
- Consultations with specialists are not required.
- Medication type: adequate analgesia, no restrictions.

Moderate risk for drug abuse calls for another layer of vigilance in addition to the routine monitoring established for low-risk patients:

- Regular follow-up visits and prescriptions refills should occur every 2 weeks initially.
- Observe patients for signs of complicating comorbid diagnoses, such as anxiety, depression, or a sleep disorder.
- Consider referring the patient for evaluation by pain management and psychiatric specialists.
- Conduct regular checks (every 6-12 months) of your state's prescription monitoring database, if available, or consult with the patient's pharmacist.
- Visit with the patient's family members or other third parties to verify the patient's accounts and for evidence of environmental influences.
- Institute random urinalysis (or another screening method) to confirm compliance with medication levels.
- Consider checking leftover medications to verify their quantity.
- Consider limiting the use of rapid-onset analgesics.

High-risk patients require the following measures of intense monitoring in addition to those required by the low-risk and moderate-risk groups:

- Schedule regular follow-up visits more frequently than usual. If problems develop, shorten the treatment interval to weekly.
- Prescribe just enough medication to last until the next appointment and ensure that prescription refills are contingent upon attendance.
- Typically, psychiatric and addiction-medicine consultations are required. Consider consultation with a pain management specialist. Coordinate treatment.
- Conduct regular urine (or other) drug screenings in addition to some unexpected screenings.
- Consider using blood screenings.
- During every visit, count the patient's leftover medication.
- Consult a prescription database (if available) more frequently.
- Strongly enforce the treatment agreement.
- Avoid prescribing rapid-onset analgesics and consider limiting short-acting analgesics.

The 3 risk categories help make treatment decisions easier but should not be used to label patients. Remember that the need to monitor for aberrant behavior is ongoing, and patients can move from 1 risk group to another throughout the course of treatment. For example, a patient initially assessed as low risk may later display multiple aberrant behaviors in response to a deteriorating physical condition or life stresses.

In general, exhibiting more than 3 mildly aberrant behaviors during 1 year or exhibiting 1 egregious behavior should cause a patient to move to a higher risk category and to be monitored more closely. If patients remain in the low-risk category for 6 months, the interval between visits and refills of medication can be increased. Eventually, when patients have remained in the low-risk category for 1 year, refills that last for 3 months are common.

Managing Patients Who Exhibit Aberrant Behaviors

Patients who begin to exhibit aberrant drug-related behaviors should be monitored more strictly than are patients who comply. The monitoring level intensifies with the frequency, severity, and persistence of the aberrant behavior. For example:

> Patty is 43 years old and has experienced chronic fatigue, fibromyalgia, and low back pain for many years. Patty's score on the Opioid Risk Tool placed her in the high-risk category for problems with managing opioid intake. Sexually molested at age 5, she was diagnosed as having bipolar disorder. Her father was a habitual cocaine user, so she grew up seeing substances abused in her childhood home. Her social life as an adult revolved around beer parties and illicit drug use, including the recreational consumption of prescription opioids. Patty began exhibiting aberrant behaviors almost immediately after she received a prescription for an opioid to manage her pain. She called the clinic frequently for unauthorized refills and missed appointments. Unauthorized prescription drugs were found in the results of a urine screening.

As a patient, Patty would require the very highest level of monitoring, including frequent visits and urine drug screenings, a referral for the management of her substance abuse and mental health, the use of a third party to monitor her prescriptions, and a possible change in her treatment to a medication less likely to be abused. Even with those safeguards, it may eventually become clear that long-term opioid therapy is not an option for Patty because of her uncontrolled opioid consumption and habits involving illicit drugs. It is also possible that her problem behavior could be curtailed, so that in her case, opioid therapy would be successful.

As previously discussed, the reasons patients misbehave may not always be rooted in addiction. Some patients do not comply because of uncontrolled pain, a psychiatric disorder, or other problems. Such motivations cannot be detected by radiographs or the results of laboratory testing. For those reasons, the monitoring process is so vital. Only by addressing any problems that arise, adjusting the treatment plan accordingly, and observing the outcome can the patient's primary problem be pinpointed and treated.

If pain is causing a patient's drug-seeking behavior, an increase in opioids to an analgesic level could halt the behavior. It is also possible that the behavior is due to a specific pain condition that is refractory to treatment with opioids. A strong indicator of a substance-use disorder is an overwhelming focus on opioids to the exclusion of any other pain therapies, which suggests that the reward sought is psychologic rather than analgesic. If the patient shows signs of ongoing abuse of a prescription opioid, some actions to consider (in addition to the high-risk monitoring strategies already outlined) include:

• Even more frequent visits with strict counts of medication.
• A stringent program of drug screening.
• The use of opioids that carry less "binge" or abuse potential.
• Enlisting a third party, usually a family member, to control and administer the patient's medications.

Medication Choices

An understanding of the patient's substance-abuse history, if one exists, can help the clinician choose the appropriate pain medication. It may be wise to avoid prescribing medications with properties similar to those of drugs abused in the past. Agents with a rapid onset of action may afford greater "binge" potential for some patients, and a pain medication with a slower onset of action, such as methadone or buprenorphine may be preferable for those individuals. It may be that the patient has problems managing the psychologic effects of opioids but also is experiencing severe pain. Opioids with a slow-release mechanism of action or a long half-life are preferred for patients with pain that must be managed with opioids but who exhibit abuse. As always, clinical decisions must be reached on an individual basis.

When used to treat pain, methadone requires more frequent dosing than the daily doses given for the treatment of addiction, but methadone should be introduced at a low dose (no higher than 30 mg daily)[11] that can be very slowly titrated higher. It is doubly vital to schedule frequent visits from the patient and counts of leftover medication to ensure compliance with all dosing directions. Regular screening of urine (or other screening measures) should be used to determine that medication is being used as prescribed and that no illicit drugs are being taken. This is particularly critical if methadone is the opioid of choice, because its long half-life may result in fatalities from drug interactions or a buildup in the system from too high an initial dose or overuse by the patient.[12]

Enlisting a Third Party

It is wise to interview family members to gain their support. Family members are a common source of complaints to medical boards; therefore, it is important that family members clearly understand and participate in the patient's goals of treatment. Sometimes, the recruitment of a family member or close friend to control and dole out the prescribed portion of medication is the right solution for a patient who cannot manage his or her own intake. Interviewing family members also provides a good opportunity to learn whether misconceptions associated with opioids are influencing the family's attitude toward the patient and possibly compromising chances for the success of treatment. Impart factual scientific information regarding the prescribing of opioids but be prepared to listen to the family's concerns. Clear communication will increase chances of gaining cooperation from the patient and from the patient's loved ones. Listening well may also help the clinician to determine whether a serious drug problem exists.

Patients with a History of Substance Abuse

Doctors and other practitioners are sometimes reluctant to treat the pain of patients with a past substance-use disorder. Is it any wonder that patients hesitate to disclose a history of substance abuse? Undertreating the pain of a former drug abuser may worsen drug-seeking behaviors. However, reexposing a patient to a substance that he or she once abused does indeed confer a risk of the recurrence of abuse. A strong focused structure for pain treatment is a must. Patients who only recently entered recovery or whose abuse history includes opiates require the most stringent monitoring of all. The only way to know whether a former abuser will respond therapeutically to opioids prescribed to treat pain is to track their response using a tool such as the Four A's. Any aberrant behaviors that occur must be rigorously monitored, addressed with the patient, and documented. The patient must demonstrate a commitment to following the parameters of the treatment plan to which he or she agreed. If the patient can do this and the clinician exercises due vigilance, opioids may be prescribed safely even in patients with a history of abusing drugs.

To plan the best treatment for pain, it is advisable to obtain all possible information (particularly the drugs of choice) about an individual's habits while he or she was abusing substances. Encourage honesty in self-reports from the patient, including the timeline of the history of drug abuse and how recently it occurred. During the reassessment that occurs during each clinic visit, it is especially important to focus on substance-abuse issues.

The patient's medical record must reflect the clinician's awareness of a prior substance-use disorder, the steps taken to address it, and the details of the current pain condition. The record must state that any prescribed opioids are being given to treat pain, not addiction.

Medication Choices

For patients with histories of drug abuse, prescribe opioids with reduced potential for abuse and consider nonpharmacologic interventions. Do not prescribe benzodiazepines or sedatives instead of analgesic medication, however, or prescribe nonpharmacologic treatments when medication is the appropriate treatment.

The measures for monitoring high-risk patients should be followed. In addition, for patients in recovery:

- Verify the patient's recovery process in a 12-step or other treatment program and understand its importance in that patient's life. Some clinicians require that a patient bring proof of ongoing participation in a recovery group to every clinic visit.
- Counsel patients to avoid social and family contacts that could influence them to resume substance abuse. Relationships may need to be adjusted to allow the patient to consume medication for pain while abstaining from abuse. The patient must understand the importance to his or her recovery of avoiding former cues to abuse and of developing a strong social and family support system.
- Explain to the patient that "liking" the experience of taking an analgesic does not mean that sobriety has been lost, as long as the drug intake is controlled. The experience should, however, prompt the patient to guard against the danger of reactivating an addiction and losing sobriety.

• Tell the patient that chronic pain is a stressful event that could trigger a recurrence of abuse. Encourage him or her to seek help and support when needed to ease the stress induced by chronic pain and to combat any drug cravings experienced.

Often, patients no one believed could be managed on opioid therapy have experienced a good outcome with the right medication adjustments and a multidisciplinary approach. If opioids cannot be safely prescribed for a given patient, however, opioid treatment may need to be discontinued. More on that subject will follow later in the chapter.

Treating Comorbid Psychiatric Disorders

Psychiatric illnesses are common in people who abuse drugs. If opioid therapy is being considered for the treatment of chronic pain in patients with a history of either a mental disorder or a substance-use disorder, both problems must be optimally managed for the best outcome.

The Substance Abuse and Mental Health Services Administration encourages an integrated approach to treatment. Patients themselves seem to have an intuitive grasp of this need. When asked, patients who exhibited both posttraumatic stress disorder and substance abuse expressed their own belief that those 2 disorders are related, and they voiced a preference to be treated simultaneously for both. Unfortunately, most people who receive treatment do so for only 1 disorder, and many more receive no treatment at all. Although an integrated treatment approach is preferred, some treatment is certainly better than no treatment. Consider the following example:

> A 24-year-old woman who was referred for the management of chronic daily headache was being treated with benzodiazepines, antidepressants, and opioids. She was diagnosed as having bipolar disease at the age of 21 years. She escalated her use of short-acting opioids without a clear improvement in function.

That case illustrates an individual who could benefit from the expertise of a psychiatrist who could treat her bipolar disorder, a neurologist who could evaluate her headaches, a psychologist to help her deal with confounding lifelong mental health problems, and an addiction specialist to prevent opioid abuse as well as medication to control pain.

The ultimate goal of pain management is to customize treatment for the individual patient, depending on his or her particular types of problems. The unfortunate truth is that healthcare systems and insurance companies rarely recognize that these illnesses are deeply intertwined and interactive. Instead, insurance providers exhibit little support for an integrated treatment approach and insist on separate delivery systems and cheap-to-nonexistent coverage and reimbursement, particularly for behavioral therapies.

When an Active Addictive Disorder Is Suspected

Some patients are more interested in obtaining opioids or other narcotics than in pain control. If it is determined that the individual is suffering from active addictive disease rather than uncontrolled pain or some other cause of aberrant behavior, that patient needs and deserves treatment for addiction. The right kind of treatment decreases drug use in abusers by 40% to 60%,[13] but patients must stay in treatment long enough for therapy to take effect.

Many types of treatment for addiction are available, and the effectiveness of a given program will vary with the individual. The NIDA[13] advises that an effective program:

- Must be readily available.
- Should address multiple needs such as the patient's medical, psychologic, social, occupational, and legal problems.
- Need not be voluntary on the part of the patient to be effective.
- Must be assessed and modified as necessary.
- Must be of adequate length (3 months is the average for achieving improvement).
- May combine medication for addiction treatment with behavioral counseling.
- Encourages participation in a 12-step or other self-help group to complement formal treatment.

The patient's well-being and clinical progress depend on finding effective treatment. Addiction is a chronic illness that may recur and require multiple treatment episodes. As with chronic pain, the commitment to treating addiction is long term. Recurrence of an addiction does not mean that drug treatment is ineffective, nor is it a reason to abandon pain management; it is a signal to intensify efforts of recovery.

Although it is possible to treat acute pain in a patient with an addictive disorder, for opioid therapy to be successful longer term, substance intake must be strictly controlled. In addition to all high-risk strategies previously mentioned, clinicians should consider instituting the following measures when managing patients who exhibit an active abuse problem:

- Clarify to the patient that the provision of medication will be stringently controlled.
- Discontinue the rescue dose for breakthrough pain.
- Explain to the patient that if he or she runs out of medication before the set refill date, no further medication will be provided without a police report documenting the theft of those drugs.
- Step up frequent urine screenings and office visits.
- Never allow the patient to miss a mandatory medication count.
- Explain that the detection of illegal substances in urine or blood will be grounds for terminating opioid therapy.
- Require nonopioid interventions such as psychotherapy and referrals to needed specialists.
- Be sure to obtain the patient's signed consent to inform any additional participating healthcare providers of his or her status as a recovering substance abuser.
- Contact all involved healthcare providers and closely coordinate care.
- Require proof from the patient of participation in all required therapies and interventions.

Patients with moderate-to-severe pain in addition to a substance-use disorder tend to gain little benefit from treatment for addiction unless the pain is controlled first. Be aware that treating pain with an opioid agonist-antagonist combination (eg, pentazocine) may cause acute withdrawal in an active abuser of morphine-type drugs. Buprenorphine is a partial agonist that can also cause withdrawal in an opioid-tolerant person by displacing the opioid from the mu receptor and occupying that receptor itself. If a patient is taking methadone for addiction treatment, the dose must be slowly increased to achieve analgesic benefits. Titrate methadone carefully and slowly and with attention to the long half-life of that drug and its potential for inducing respiratory depression. If methadone is not used for pain control, another medication should be prescribed to relieve pain in addition to the daily dose of methadone for treatment of opioid addiction.

Patients who have difficulty taking opioids safely should learn to take a strong partnership role in their own pain-management program while preventing the recurrence of substance abuse. If these patients can be directed to programs with other members who also suffer from chronic pain and addiction, the support and validation they receive there can be invaluable.

Remember, however, that some patients may need to discontinue opioid therapy. This is warranted if the patient's noncompliance is severely disrupting opioid therapy and trust cannot be reestablished. Perhaps the acid test is to determine whether opioid therapy is making the patient's life better or worse. The patient who may be a poor candidate for opioid therapy is the one whose physical functioning, quality of life, social and family interactions, and professional life are characterized by marked and continuing deterioration. If patients are using prescription medications to escape from life rather than to participate more fully in it, opioids are probably the wrong treatment.

It is not a failure to terminate a treatment that is harmful and ineffective. As with any other medical treatment, it is poor practice to continue a therapy that demonstrates a clear

---

Box VI:4 **Exit Strategy to Discontinue Opioid Therapy**

- Meet with the patient.
- Review the exit criteria agreed to in the treatment agreement.
- Clarify that the termination of opioid treatment is for the patient's benefit.
- Clarify that exiting opioid therapy is not synonymous with abandoning pain management.
- Consider tapering opioids gradually over 1 month.
- Implement nonopioid pain strategies, including psychiatric or behavioral therapy; physical therapy; treatment with nonopioid analgesics; treatment for insomnia, anxiety, or depression; or interventional procedures.

If the patient does not cooperate with the plan for outpatient tapering of the prescribed medication:

- Do not provide additional opioids.
- Refer the patient to either an inpatient program or a comprehensive outpatient program for opioid discontinuation.
- Provide nonopioid medical maintenance until the patient is admitted to the next phase of his or her treatment.

If addiction is the problem, refer the patient for addiction management or co-management.

lack of benefit for the individual. Terminating treatment with an opioid is not tantamount to abandoning pain management. Remember that the well-being of a patient is not synonymous with unrestricted access to opioids.

Discontinuing Opioid Therapy

If adverse effects of opioid therapy are severe, ongoing, and threaten to submerge a patient's life in chaos despite clinical interventions, it may be time to consider a cessation of opioids. Be aware that withdrawal from opioids can produce temporary hyperalgesia. In 1 study, 10 patients whose pain condition had stabilized as a result of treatment with controlled-release morphine were subjected to the abrupt cessation of opioids through the administration of a placebo.[14] These nonaddicted patients did not display drug craving but did experience pain that disrupted activity, mood, relationships, sleep, and enjoyment of life.

Explain the effect of temporarily heightened pain to the patient and be prepared to help manage it or to make referrals. To taper opioid treatment in a patient who might otherwise experience abstinence syndrome is compassionate and ethical practice. See Box VI:4 for a suggested exit strategy.

The chapter that is devoted to legal issues in opioid prescribing includes a more extensive discussion of the legal and ethical responsibilities expected of a clinician when a patient's opioid therapy must be withdrawn. A clinician is not obligated to put his or her own practice at risk by continuing to provide opioids to a chronic abuser.

Drug Screening: Checking for Compliance

Trust is a necessary component of the clinician-patient relationship, but research indicates it is unwise to depend on a patient's word alone that drugs are being consumed as prescribed. In a study of 33,000 patients treated with oxycodone, 35% failed to show the expected medication concentration in a check of urine samples.[15] In a smaller investigation in which pain patients' statements about their drug consumption were measured against the actual results of toxicologic urine screenings, the patients' statements matched their test results only 68% of the time.[16]

Although noncompliance is common in patients who are prescribed opioids, it does not always reach the level that threatens the integrity of the therapy. Noncompliance can even be the sign of a patient's confusion in juggling multiple medications. Nonetheless, noncompliance is a serious clinical event that must be addressed.

The high degree of noncompliance with treatment for drug abuse is a reason to screen for appropriate drug levels, particularly among patients at highest risk for using opioids nonmedically. Some patients undergoing treatment for drug abuse will show no other signs of problematic behavior.[17] A drug screening should be approached as a consensual diagnostic test, as part of the treatment agreement, and as a factor of mutual benefit to the patient and the clinician. In the same way that analysis of the glucose level is essential to diabetic patients (to ensure that treatment is effective), drug screening is essential to opioid-treated patients.

A great difference exists between the standards and needs of forensic testing for legal use and clinical testing. The purpose of forensic testing is usually to look for a discrepancy, and clinical testing seeks to establish compliance. Forensic testing is governed by strict rules about the chain of custody that are difficult to implement in a medical setting. A sample collected in a clinic is usually insufficient for a legal decision.

Among other benefits, clinical drug screening can:

- Serve as a deterrent to inappropriate drug taking.
- Provide objective evidence of abstinence from drugs of abuse.
- Monitor the response to treatment.
- Assist with the diagnosis.
- Provide advocacy for a patient by demonstrating compliance to such interested parties as family members, law-enforcement authorities, and employers.
- Demonstrate to regulatory authorities a clinician's dedication to monitoring patients.
- Support a clinician's medical decisions.

Who should be tested? Ideally, all patients who begin opioid therapy for the first time for pain should be tested. New patients who are already undergoing treatment with a controlled substance should also be screened. Testing is recommended when aberrant behavior is suspected or confirmed, when changes in treatment are being made, when pain persists despite aggressive treatment, and to provide support for the referral of a patient for substance-abuse assessment.

Drug testing, though a valuable tool, is subject to various drawbacks, often imposed by the limits of technology and by human error.

- Available tests are not sensitive enough to detect the presence or amount of many substances.
- False-positive and false-negative results are common, as is the misinterpretation of results.
- Drug screening results are influenced by many factors, including the equipment and methods used by a particular laboratory, the characteristics of the drug, and the peculiarities of drug metabolism in individual patients.
- During an investigation by regulatory or legal authorities, clinicians may be questioned about the reasons a patient was not discharged after drug screening results revealed an illicit drug.

Before ordering a drug screening, be sure the patient's medical record accurately reflects all medications that the patient is currently taking. It is helpful to talk with the patient; consider asking point-blank whether he or she expects the screening to reveal any unauthorized substances. Explain that drug testing is part of the effort to monitor the clinical efficacy of treatment and is not a game of "gotcha." Positive or problematic results are cues to counsel the patient, to tighten treatment boundaries, and (possibly) to refer that individual for substance-abuse treatment. The clinician should:

- Discuss any unexpected results with the laboratory.
- Schedule an appointment with the patient to discuss his or her results.
- Use those results to enhance the clinician-patient relationship and to encourage positive change.
- Document all results, their interpretation, and the steps taken to address them in the patient's medical chart.

Encourage the patient to talk about what has occurred. The presence of unauthorized substances may not be reason enough to halt therapy outright, and any positive results of drug screening must be considered within the total context of the Four A's.

For Which Drugs Should Pain Management Clinicians Screen?

The patient should be tested for the presence of all prescribed drugs and for standard opioids such as hydrocodone, oxycodone, and hydromorphone. At a minimum, benzodiazepines should also be included because they are often revealed in the results of toxicology reports of overdose deaths associated with opioid use. The unauthorized presence of benzodiazepines should spur a reappraisal of treatment and possibly a referral for the treatment of a psychologic disorder or substance-abuse problems.

The following substances may be of interest to a pain-control provider:

- Amphetamines or methamphetamine.
- Anticonvulsant medications.
- Barbiturates.
- Benzodiazepines.
- Cocaine.
- Marijuana (tetrahydrocannabinol).
- Methylphenidate.
- Opiates, including:
    Codeine.
    Diacetylmorphine.
    Dihydrocodeine.
    Fentanyl.
    Hydrocodone.
    Meperidine.
    Methadone.
    Morphine.
    Oxymorphone.
    Oxycodone.
    Propoxyphene.
    Tramadol.
- Phencyclidine.
- Tricyclic medications.
- Ethanol.

The decision of whether to screen for illegal drugs (and if so, for which ones) must be made by the clinician. We have already seen that an abuser of street drugs is at increased risk for abusing prescription medications, so some degree of screening for illicit substances is advised. Some clinicians choose not to screen for tetrahydrocannabinol, which, though illegal to most users, may have some clinical benefit, but they do screen for cocaine, a drug with no clinical use. Others, mindful of the risks of polysubstance abuse, screen for the presence of any illegal drugs. A patient who displays a pattern of illegal substance abuse must seek treatment for a substance-use disorder. Continued failure to comply is grounds for the cessation of opioid therapy.

Methods of Detection: A Comparison

The main biochemical measures used to detect drug use are: urine, blood, saliva, perspiration, and (more recently and less commonly) hair analysis. Different methods confer various limitations and advantages related to the ease of use, degree of invasiveness, cost, and window of detection (the interval between the ingestion of a drug and the beginning of excretion of that drug and its metabolites at a concentration above a test cutoff score).

- Blood (or serum) testing is very effective in detecting low levels of substances but is an invasive and expensive procedure with a window of detection that is limited to current drug use only.
- Oral fluid (saliva) collection has the second shortest detection window (up to 4 hours) after serum testing and offers the advantages of easy collection and limited invasiveness. However, drugs and metabolites are generally retained in saliva at lower levels than those found in urine. Saliva testing is a new method that is increasing in popularity.
- Hair analysis can have a window of detection of up to 6 months. However, some have claimed that hair testing involves a racial bias because dark hair binds more easily to certain drugs than does fair or gray hair. The testing of hair is somewhat cumbersome to perform and is prone to providing a false-negative result. It is usually inefficient for clinical testing.
- The window of detection for drugs in perspiration is up to 1 week. Perspiration is gathered over several days or weeks by means of a patch that is rather inefficient in the detection of drug use for pain management and is better suited to monitoring drug use in patients participating in a chemical dependency program.
- The most useful and widespread clinical tool used to test for compliance is urine screening. Less expensive and invasive than serum testing, urine screening offers a window of detection ranging from 12 to 72 hours, ease of collection, and a good method of detecting drug metabolites. Urine screening is used in most compliance testing, but saliva testing may become more common because of several characteristics that recommend it for clinical use.

Urine Toxicology Screening

Screening the urine for the presence of prescribed opioids and the absence of unauthorized drugs is valuable for the safe management of the pain patient. If a history of substance abuse exists, urine screening can enable the clinician to diagnose and address the early recurrence of drug misuse. It also helps keep boundaries firmly in sight and reinforces the integrity of the treatment plan agreed to by the provider and the patient. These are significant advantages.

A patient will exhibit a problematic test result from a urine screening when:

- Illicit drugs are present.
- Prescription drugs that were not prescribed are present.
- The opioids prescribed are not present (which could indicate hoarding the medication,

binging that causes the patient to run out of medication early, or diverting the medication for sale).

The available testing measures have a high degree of reliability, but the results must be interpreted with caution.

Types of Urine Screening

Most effective urine screenings consist of 2 steps: an initial screening and a confirmation. The initial screening is usually performed by means of either a radioactive or enzyme-mediated immunoassay test that reveals whether substances are present. Two less commonly used forms of immunoassays are the fluorescence polarization and the particle immunoassay. Immunoassays can be used to screen for most classes of drugs or their metabolites but typically do not isolate specific opioids. Positive test results should be confirmed by a second test. The gold standard for confirmation testing is the gas chromatography/mass spectrometry (GC/MS) test, which is highly specific and sensitive. The GC/MS detects the actual molecular structure of the drug and its metabolites. It uses 2 techniques: chromatography procedures to separate the various components and mass spectrometry to identify specific components of the specimen. This test must be performed in a laboratory. High-performance liquid chromatography is another chromatographic method of specific drug identification that is faster and less expensive than a GC/MS. However, the GC/MS is considered the legal standard and is recommended if legal consequences are of concern.

The 5 basic drugs (amphetamines, cocaine, opiates, marijuana, and phencyclidine) that are included in the initial screening are sometimes called the "Federal Five." A routine immunoassay does not include benzodiazepines or barbiturates and will not likely identify oxycodone or fentanyl. The testing for those drugs must be requested specifically from most laboratories. Tests for methadone and buprenorphine also are available.

Most "windows" for the detection of drugs via urine immunoassay screenings are about 1 to 3 days (Box VI:5). Exceptions include screening for tetrahydrocannabinol, which can

Box VI:5	**Detection Windows for Immunoassay Urine Screening**
Amphetamines	1 - 4 d
Barbiturates	Up to 6 d (up to 30 d after phenobarbital)
Cocaine	2 - 3 d (7 d for heavy or long-term use, possibly longer)
Methadone	2 - 3 d
Opiates	2 - 4 d (heroin metabolite 6-monoacetylmorphine < 8 h)
Marijuana	Up to 5 d for occasional use (30 d for long-term use, sometimes longer)
Benzodiazepines	Up to 7 d (up to 30 d for diazepam and chlordiazepoxide)
Propoxyphene	Up to 7 d
Phencyclidine	2 - 7 d (up to 14 d for long-term use)
Ethanol	6 to 10 h (occasionally longer)
Lysergic acid diethylamide	Up to 5 d

Material provided by Dominion Diagnostics. 211 Circuit Drive, North Kingstown, RI 02852.

linger for a month or more in long-term users, and benzodiazepines, which, when abused in large quantities, can take weeks to eliminate depending on the amount and type ingested.

Testing should be performed for suspected alcohol abuse, which can compromise the safety and efficacy of opioid treatment in several ways. One adverse effect of alcohol is to hasten the action of sustained-release opioid formulations. The presence of glucose can confound testing for alcohol abuse because urine that contains glucose can produce ethanol. If glucose is found in an ethanol-positive specimen, the ethanol may have been caused by the fermentation of a sample that was not properly refrigerated. A specific test for an exclusive metabolite of ethanol can alleviate this concern but is probably worthwhile only when heavy alcohol consumption is suspected.

Many standard drug-testing packages are based on workplace requirements rather than on clinical needs. Drug testing in the workplace is governed by federal guidelines published by the US Department of Health and Human Services and codified by the Department of Transportation. The federal guidelines outline specific requirements, such as those for split specimens, and also require that trained medical review officers interpret the results. Workplace measures such as split specimens usually are not needed in clinical settings, but clinical guidelines are still incomplete. For instance, although medical review officers are not required in clinical settings, it is best to give all staff who collect and handle specimens the best training available.

Most immunoassay testing can be performed at the point of care (POC) if the available clinical facilities allow. POC devices vary in quality, cutoff scores, and methods of reading results. It is advisable to select a device that has been approved by the FDA. POC testing is cost-effective and provides quicker results than do most laboratories. POC devices cannot handle all the testing needs for patients treated for pain, however, because testing for a wider range of drugs or a confirmation such as a GC/MS must be performed by a laboratory.

Laboratory testing has several important advantages, including extensive training of personnel, a formalized chain of custody for handling the sample, a high degree of accuracy, and the availability of tests for specific substances. It is wise to cultivate a relationship with a testing laboratory, understand the procedures of that service, and make your own needs clear to the laboratory staff.

Laboratory Methods of Urine Testing

Different laboratories may use different methods of performing urine screenings. Clinicians should know the operating procedure of the chosen laboratory. In particular, one should ask the lab professionals:

• Which drugs are identified by the tests available?
• What are the cutoff scores that are used to judge positive or negative results?

If the clinician knows which drugs he or she would like to test for, it may be necessary to request those results from the laboratory. In addition, not every laboratory will automatically send a positive immunoassay sample for a confirmatory GC/MS test. It may be necessary to request that this be done.

Typically, the cutoff scores set by laboratories are dictated by industry and government needs. Clinicians should either instruct laboratories where to set cutoff scores or ask them to eliminate the cutoff scores altogether. For clinical purposes, cutoffs usually are not needed;

it is more important to know whether or not the drug is present. Furthermore, certain opioids may not be detected if cutoff scores are set too high because molecules sufficient for detection are not present. It is usually advisable to request that laboratories test samples to the limits of detection, because any amount of substance is likely to be of concern.

Urine Specimen Validity

A minority of patients will try to tamper with the urine sample. Samples of an unusual color, an unusually small sample size, or a sample that is too hot or too cold to the touch should be discussed with the patient. The urine sample should be sent to the laboratory as soon as possible. If it is not sent immediately, it should be refrigerated until it is shipped. Specimens should be received by a laboratory within 7 days after collection. Urine contains the following substances that can be used to determine whether specimens are valid and consistent with human urine:[18]

- Creatinine: This product of muscle contraction is released into urine at a fairly constant rate and serves as an indicator of hydration. The normal range for creatinine is 20 to 400 mg/dL. A level of less than 20 mg/dL could indicate excessive drinking or dilution of the sample with a substance such as water. A creatinine level of less than 5 mg/dL is inconsistent with human urine.
- Specific gravity: As substances are added to urine, specific gravity increases; therefore, the greater the concentration, the greater the specific gravity. A normal range for specific gravity is from 1.003 to 1.030, and a specific gravity of 1.000 is practically water.
- pH: A pH value outside the normal range of 4.5 to 9.0 could indicate adulteration of the sample. Several commercial adulterants (nitrates and chromate, which work principally by foiling the confirmation testing) are sold online and in magazines and shops devoted to recreational drug use.
- Temperature: The temperature of a urine sample should range from 90°F to 100°F within 4 minutes of voiding. Therefore, temperature strips affixed to the sample cup should be read within 4 minutes (or the temperature should be otherwise measured). If the temperature strip does not register a value, the specimen should be rechecked immediately; a new cup should be used and the results should be recorded.

Interpreting the Results of Urine Screening

The greatest concern in the use of urine screenings is that they may be misinterpreted. Metabolic properties of the patient can contribute to the likelihood of misinterpretation, and clerical or clinical error can cause a false result. However, even apparently straightforward results are not always easy to interpret. If, for example, the results of the screening fail to show the expected level of prescribed opioids, the clinician will not know whether the patient took all the medication early because of uncontrolled pain, sold some or all of the medication, or other factors influenced the test results. Professional "diverters" often take enough medication before visits to ensure appropriate test results. Urine drug screening is useful only in conjunction with a focus on the Four A's and other monitoring measures that highlight the individual. Factors that can influence results include:

• Urine pH.
• Urine volume.
• Body weight.
• The presence or absence of malabsorption.
• Concurrent medications.
• The pharmacokinetic properties of the drug.
• The amount of the drug ingested.
• The route of administration.
• Dosage intervals.
• How effectively the patient can metabolize the drug.
• The duration of treatment with the medication.

This list illustrates the limitations of urine testing. It is a good tool, and even the knowledge that the test will be performed can increase patient compliance, but the results are not always 100% accurate and can be misleading. A positive result from a urine screening does not provide enough information on drug use to establish exposure time, dose, and frequency of drug use. Nor does a positive test result provide enough information to diagnose drug addiction, physical dependence, or impairment.

Metabolic Issues and Drug Detection in Urine
The metabolic influences on drug detection are of 2 different types:

• The properties and distribution of the drug.
• Individual variations in the metabolic rate of patients.

Some substances are detected in urine because they are metabolites of the consumed drug or because they are byproducts of the commercial manufacturing process (Box VI:6). Thus it should be understood that small amounts of these secondary drug metabolites do not necessarily mean that an unauthorized opioid has been ingested.
For example:

• Codeine is metabolized to morphine and is partially metabolized to hydrocodone.
• Hydrocodone can cause a positive result from tests for the metabolite hydromorphone.
• Some evidence indicates morphine can produce the minor metabolite hydromorphone.[19]

The confirmation of a test result via a GC/MS is important in pain management because heroin and codeine are both metabolized to morphine. A routine immunoassay will detect the presence of morphine but cannot isolate its source without a follow-up GC/MS. Heroin is particularly difficult to detect in the results of a urine screening because it begins to metabolize into morphine in a matter of minutes. A metabolite that definitely indicates the presence of heroin, 6-monoacetylmorphine, is rarely revealed in the results of a urine screening because it dissipates so quickly.
The peculiarities of drug metabolites can also skew test results. False-positive results for amphetamines have been blamed on certain diet pills, such as chlobenzorex and

fenproporex, or on the use of an over-the-counter nasal inhaler containing l-methamphetamine. One infamous type of true positive can be caused by the poppy seeds found in baked goods. Poppy seeds can contain from 2 to 294 micrograms of morphine per gram and from 0.4 to 57 micrograms of codeine per gram. Concentrations in the urine peak within 3 to 8 hours but can linger up to 50 hours after ingestion. It is probably a good idea for patients undergoing regular or random urine screenings to forego poppy seeds.

False-negative results occur as well, and the amount of a substance found in the blood or urine is not always indicative of the amount ingested. Patients may metabolize a drug rapidly; this can result in a false-negative result for a drug that should be present. It is also possible that a test from a particular laboratory is not sensitive enough to detect the presence of the drug.

The adjustment of creatinine values is a procedure that is helpful in monitoring drug concentrations in the urine over time. (The ratio is the concentration of the drug, divided by the creatinine level, multiplied by 100). This is particularly advantageous for detecting the true presence of tetrahydrocannabinol, which dissipates slowly from the body. Sometimes, variations in creatinine values can be caused by changes in urine concentration. When the patient awakes, for example, his or her urine can be highly concentrated. Drinking a large amount of water can dilute the urine and influence test results. Adjustment of the value of creatinine, a metabolite that is constant, normalizes the drug level.

A patient who had been a long-term user of marijuana had a result of 83 ng/mL of that drug from an initial drug test. The following month, the test result was 57 ng/mL, and the next month, the result was 43 ng/mL. It appeared that the drug was dissipating from the patient's system and that

---

Box VI:6	Urinary Analytes for Patients Treated with an Opiate-Based Medication

*Metabolite.
† Potential impurity of commercial manufacturing.

Drug	Urinary Analytes
Morphine	Morphine Hydromorphone* Codeine†
Codeine	Codeine Morphine* Hydrocodone*
Hydrocodone	Hydrocodone Hydromorphone* 6-Hydrocodol (the stereoisomer of dihydrocodeine)
Oxycodone	Oxycodone Oxymorphone* Hydrocodone†

Material provided by Dominion Diagnostics. 211 Circuit Drive, North Kingstown, RI 02852.

compliance was being achieved. When the test results from the fourth month were read, the level of marijuana had increased again to 58 ng/mL. It appeared the patient was ingesting an unauthorized substance. However, when the laboratory adjusted the patient's creatinine levels, which revealed a high urine concentration in the fourth test, it was discovered that the level of tetrahydrocannabinol had actually decreased.

As a clinical monitoring tool, urine drug screenings confer significant benefits as long as the limitations in interpreting results are well understood. Drug screening should be applied to all patients who begin opioid therapy, and the results should spur clinical discussion, not fear and concealment.

Oral Fluid Testing

Oral fluid detection may be a more sensitive method of identifying drugs than has been generally believed. It is particularly effective in the detection of recent drug use, and it reveals both parent drugs and metabolites. Oral fluid is readily accessible and is more difficult for the patient to manipulate than urine, and collection can easily be observed. Problems with oral testing include the brief window of viability of the samples and the influence of pH on results. Rinsing the mouth with an acidic solution before testing can decrease the amount of drug detected. Oral detection is most effective when saliva has not been diluted, a factor that can be manipulated by the patient by, for example, opening the mouth wide to stimulate more saliva production. In fact, it is somewhat difficult to collect "unstimulated" saliva because jaw movement stimulates the production of saliva. Specimen collection is accomplished by having the patient spit with or without stimulation or by the use of a collection technique such as absorption or swabbing, draining, or suction. A comparison study of the effectiveness of oral fluid testing versus urine testing found a "remarkable similarity" in the pattern and frequency of positive drug test results in the general workforce.[20]

Prescription Monitoring Programs

Twenty-seven states were operating some form of prescription-monitoring program (PMP) as of 2006, and additional states are developing those programs. To varying degrees, these state programs:

- Collect prescribing and dispensing data from pharmacies.
- Review and analyze the data.
- Make those data available to healthcare practitioners, law-enforcement authorities, and regulatory agencies.

However, the circumstances under which information is available vary among the states, and not all PMPs make data available to practitioners. This state-by-state design is likely to continue. The recent passage of a national law to approve prescription-monitoring programs in all states does not provide a framework other than requiring states to share information.

A prescription monitoring database is a valuable tool with which physicians can check the drug history of a patient. Frequent checks, particularly in high-risk patients, can reveal

Box VI:7

Monitoring David: A Case Study in Comorbid Disorders

David, a 34-year-old police officer:
- Was referred to a pain clinic to manage the pain from multiple operations for a neuroma of the foot.
- Has a comorbid anxiety disorder.

David exhibited multiple and ongoing aberrant behaviors by:
- Taking prescriptions too quickly.
- Calling early for refills.
- Claiming that he lost medications.

Steps taken to increase the monitoring of David:
- Adjusted his medication.
- Requested more reports from the prescription monitoring system.
- Refused refills until the specified time.
- Scheduled more frequent (weekly) visits.
- Checked his urine and blood for the presence of prescribed medications and illicit substances.
- Referred him for substance-abuse counseling.
- Referred him to a therapist to learn coping mechanisms.
- Checked for corrective behavior.

Disagreements with David over medications continued. Nothing appeared to work, and the prescribing clinician began to feel uncomfortable working with this patient.

Finally, effective interventions were found:

- A third party, David's mother, was brought in to monitor and administer his medication.
- An effective medication to treat David's anxiety was found, and that reduced his need to seek additional unauthorized substances.

Outcome: David began to take his medications as prescribed and to present negative results from urine and blood screenings.

whether or not "doctor shopping" (obtaining opioids from several medical sources) is occurring. See the chapter on legal issues for more detail on PMPs.

Conclusion

The case study shown in Box VI:7 illustrates the complex differential presented by aberrant behaviors; and it shows the benefit of monitoring each patient individually until a workable solution that addresses pain control and proper medication use is found. Good monitoring involves all the steps outlined to this point. Clinicians should:

- Be familiar with the individual risk factors for opioid abuse.
- Screen new patients during the initial clinic visit and use clinically validated assessments to evaluate, diagnose, and possibly predict abuse or addiction in patients.
- Set the level of monitoring appropriate to the degree of risk demonstrated by each patient.
- Watch for and document any aberrant drug-related behavior that may be associated with abuse or addiction.
- Reassess each patient at frequent intervals. Every visit should include some degree of reassessment. The importance of this step cannot be overemphasized.
- Never make judgments before an appropriate assessment has been performed. Do not assume that a high-risk patient will always abuse opioids or that a low-risk patient will never do so.

References

1. Probes LM. Opioid blood levels in chronic pain management. Practical Pain Management. Apr 2005; 5(3):12-18.
2. American Academy of Pain Medicine and American Pain Society. The use of opioids for the treatment of chronic pain: a consensus statement. Glenview, IL; 1997.
3. Passik SD, Kirsh KL, Whitcomb L, Schein JR, Kaplan MA, Dodd SL, Kleinman L, Katz NP, Portenoy RK. Monitoring outcomes during long-term opioid therapy for noncancer pain: results with the Pain Assessment and Documentation Tool. J Opioid Manag 2005 Nov-Dec;1(5):257-66.
4. Bolen J. Retaining legal counsel: an attorney's perspective. The 23rd annual meeting of the American Academy of Pain Medicine. New Orleans, LA; February 7-10, 2007.
5. Fishbain DA, Cutler RB, Rosomoff HL, Rosomoff RS. Are opioid-dependent/tolerant patients impaired in driving-related skills? A structured evidence-based review. J Pain Symptom Manage. 2003 Jun;25(6):559-77.
6. Fishman SM, Bandman TB, Edwards A, Borsook D. The opioid contract in the management of chronic pain. J Pain Symptom Manage. 1999 Jul;18(1):27-37.
7. Passik SD, Weinreb HJ. Managing chronic nonmalignant pain: overcoming obstacles to the use of opioids. Adv Ther. 2000 Mar-Apr;17(2):70-83.
8. Passik SD, Kirsh KL, Whitcomb L, Portenoy RK, Katz NP, Kleinman L, Dodd SL, Schein JR. A new tool to assess and document pain outcomes in chronic pain patients receiving opioid therapy. Clin Ther. 2004 Apr;26(4):552-61.
9. American Chronic Pain Association. ACPA Medications & Chronic Pain Supplement 2007. American Chronic Pain Association: Rocklin, CA; 2007.
10. Gourlay DL, Heit HA, Almahrezi A. Universal precautions in pain medicine: a rational approach to the treatment of chronic pain. Pain Med. 2005 Mar-Apr;6(2):107-12.
11. FDA Public Health Advisory: Methadone use for pain control may result in death and life-threatening changes in breathing and heart beat. US Food and Drug Administration, US Department of Health and Human Services. Available at: http://www.fda.gov/cder/drug/advisory/methadone.htm. Accessed April 9, 2007.

12. Webster LR. Methadone-related deaths. J Opioid Manag 2005 Sep-Oct;1(4):211-7.

13. National Institute on Drug Abuse, National Institutes of Health, US Department of Health and Human Services. Principles of drug addiction treatment: a research-based guide. NIH Publication No. 00-4180. Rockville, MD. Printed October 1999, Reprinted July 2000.

14. Cowan DT, Wilson-Barnett DJ, Griffiths P, Vaughan DJA, Gondhia A, Allan LG. A randomized, double-blind, placebo-controlled, cross-over pilot study to assess the effects of long-term opioid drug consumption and subsequent abstinence in chronic non-cancer pain patients receiving controlled-release morphine. Pain Med. 2005 Mar-Apr; 6(2):113-21.

15. Pembrook L. Two screening tests scrutinize urine, identify noncompliant patients. Pain Medicine News. 2005; August 10.

16. Berndt S, Maier C, Schutz HW. Polymedication and medication compliance in patients with chronic non-malignant pain. Pain. 1993 Mar;52(3):331-9.

17. Katz NP, Sherburne S, Beach M, Rose RJ, Vielguth J, Bradley J, Fanciullo GJ. Behavioral monitoring and urine toxicology testing in patients receiving long-term opioid therapy. Anesth Analg. 2003 Oct;97(4):1097-102, table of contents.

18. Dominion Diagnostics. 211 Circuit Drive, North Kingstown, RI 02852. Available at: http//:www.dominiondiagnostics.com. Accessed April 10, 2007.

19. Cone EJ, Heit HA, Caplan YH, Gourlay D. Evidence of morphine metabolism to hydromorphone in pain patients chronically treated with morphine. J Anal Toxicol 2006 Jan-Feb;30(1):1-5.

20. Cone EJ, Presley L, Lehrer M, Seiter W, Smith M, Kardos KW, Fritch D, Salamone S, Niedbala RS. Oral fluid testing for drugs of abuse: positive prevalence rates by Intercept immunoassay screening and GC-MS-MS confirmation and suggested cutoff concentrations. J Anal Toxicol. 2002 Nov-Dec;26(8):541-6.

21. American Academy of Pain Medicine. Long-term controlled substances therapy for chronic pain: sample agreement. A consent form from the American Academy of Pain Medicine Web site. Available at: http://www.painmed.org/productpub/statements/pdfs/controlled_substances_sample_a grmt.pdf. Accessed April 10, 2007.

CHAPTER VII

LEGAL ISSUES OF OPIOID PRESCRIBING

Doing what's right isn't the problem. It's knowing what's right.
- Lyndon B. Johnson, former US President[1]

Strict regulations govern the prescribing of opioids and other controlled substances (CS). Most clinicians are more than willing to comply with all the expectations that accompany long-term opioid therapy. That, however, is no simple task. Many physicians and other practitioners are not familiar with the applicable laws, guidelines, and policies. Even when they know the rules, those rules can change or undergo a fresh interpretation that throws doubt on accepted legal standards.

This chapter summarizes the legal ramifications of prescribing opioids. It reviews state and federal laws, the role of regulatory agencies, the pros and cons of prescription-monitoring databases, the questions surrounding the discharging of noncompliant patients, and many other issues. The steps outlined are designed to protect the practice of any prescribing clinician via meticulous recordkeeping and adherence to all regulations, insofar as they are currently understood. Of primary importance is the section calling for new partnerships among clinicians, drug regulators, law-enforcement officials, and pharmacists. The dual goal of all interested parties is to fight nonmedical opioid use and to ensure that patients do not suffer pain because of needless barriers to treatment.

Balancing Good Law and Good Medicine

Laws, like standards of physical beauty, change with the times. In the late 19th century, heroin was introduced (first as a powerful cough suppressant and then as a long-awaited and legal "cure" for morphine addiction). The US federal government first began regulating the sale and distribution of CS in 1914 with passage of the Harrison Act. In 1961, the era of global drug control was under way, and the Single Convention on Narcotic Drugs, an international treaty against illicit drug manufacturing and trafficking, was created. Over the next decade, a wider social acceptance of drug experimentation and an increase in drug-related street violence spurred the US government to enact stricter drug control. In 1970, Congress consolidated existing drug laws into 1 extensive regulatory and enforcement instrument: the Controlled Substances Act (CSA).

Today, the opiate-based medications needed to relieve pain are prescribed under tight control. The network of laws, regulations, policies, and guidelines that govern opioids and other CS are far-reaching and complex. Some doctors chafe under the special strictures and maintain that no other medications – no matter how high the risk associated with their use – are the focus of such exacting government scrutiny. Regardless, medically prescribed CS are associated with special ill effects; therefore, government oversight will not diminish in the foreseeable future.

When prescribing opioids, clinicians in the United States must answer to 2 simultaneously governing structures: the federal system and the state system. Whenever federal law differs from state law, the more stringent of the 2 rules applies. See Box VII:1 for the Framework of Controlled-Substance Law in the United States.

The following definitions may be helpful. Statutes and acts passed by legislative bodies carry the force of law. Regulations are rules written by government agencies to explain the law and, as such, are enforced as law. In addition, government agencies issue policy statements, guidelines, and position statements. These are not laws but may take on the force of law if introduced as evidence in court. Familiarity with state and federal requirements is a necessity for any prescriber of opioids, beginning where the regulation of all drug traffic began: at the federal level.

Federal Law: Opioid Prescribing

It is crucial to note that no US federal law prohibits the use of opioids for analgesia. Rather, it is US policy to prevent drug abuse and diversion and to ensure that opioids are available for medical and scientific needs. Opioids and other CS approved by the FDA are part of accepted medical practice within appropriate treatment guidelines. A chronic-pain patient is specifically protected as a lawful recipient of opioid therapy and is described as "a person with intractable pain, in which no relief or cure is possible or none has been found after a reasonable effort."[2]

The Controlled Substances Act

The CSA is the bedrock of the US government's enforcement effort against drug abuse. It is also designed to protect access to CS for legitimate purposes. It regulates the manufacture, distribution, and dispensing of substances (eg, opioids and other classes of narcotics, stimulants, depressants, hallucinogens, anabolic steroids, and many chemicals used to produce illicit drugs) that are controlled because they are subject to abuse or have the potential to cause physical or psychologic dependence.

As written, US federal law could be described as "friendly" to the use of treatment with opioids to alleviate chronic pain. Federal law neither limits the quantity of opioids to be prescribed nor restricts treatment with those drugs to administration in short-term or immediate settings. This would appear to allow for the high quantities of opioids that are routinely consumed by the opioid-tolerant chronic-pain patient. However, state laws are frequently stricter, and several states do limit the size, frequency, or duration of opioid prescriptions for pain. In that case, the law of the home state trumps the less restrictive federal law.

The CSA also defines an addict as a habitual user of narcotics who endangers public morals, health, safety or welfare or who has lost self-control. Although that definition is far from ideal (for instance, it fails to distinguish between physiologic dependence and the neurobiologic disease of addiction), it does not equate the habitual opioid consumption of the chronic-pain patient with the out-of-control drug use of an addicted person.

Under the CSA, the US government:

• Recognizes the medical value of CS, including opioids.
• Appoints the Department of Health and Human Services to oversee medical and scientific decisions made in the pursuit of drug control.
• Creates a closed distribution system for CS.

- Provides for quotas to ensure sufficient supplies of CS for medical and scientific needs.
- Sets the parameters for the prescribing and practice-based use of CS.
- Describes registration and recordkeeping requirements.
- Provides for the tracking of CS.
- Sets the penalties for the nonmedical use of CS.
- Creates drug schedules I through V (or "CI" through "CV") in keeping with each drug's clinical utility and potential for abuse.
- Fights the abuse and diversion of CS.
- Is not intended to interfere with medical practice or to dictate medical decision making.

Box VII:1   **The Framework of Controlled-Substance Law**

Federal
- The Controlled Substances Act of 1970 defines what is legal in the prescribing, administering, dispensing, and distribution of controlled substances.
- The United States Code, Title 21, §§ 801-971, outlines the tenets of the Controlled Substances Act.
- The Code of Federal Regulations, Title 21, §§1300-1316, lists the specifics of controlled substances law.
- The Drug Enforcement Administration enforces the law.
- The Food and Drug Administration administers the Federal Food, Drug and Cosmetic Act, which lists the drugs considered safe, effective, and available to market.

State
- Statutes and regulations vary from state to state.
- States enforce their own controlled-substances laws, which may be stricter than federal law but will not be more lenient.
- Medical boards set the standard for medical care and professional practice.
- State agencies license healthcare professionals and maintain medical practice standards.

Drug Schedules

The schedules created by the CSA classify drugs from the most to the least harmful. Schedule I contains the drugs with the most addiction potential, which, having no acknowledged medical value, are not prescribable. Schedule V is reserved for drugs with the least addiction potential. Schedule II (CII) medications, which include opioids, have a high potential for abuse and are subject to tight control.

The Code of Federal Regulations

Clinicians who administer and prescribe opioids and other CS will find all the specifics of federal law listed in the Code of Federal Regulations (CFR), Title 21 §§1300-1316. In general, to comply with law, a prescription for an opioid must be issued:

- For a legitimate medical purpose.
- In the course of professional practice.[3]

Additional regulations address:
- Who must register with the federal government to prescribe or administer opioids.
- Which records and reports are due from registrants.
- All the rules governing prescribing and dispensing practices.
- A list of the substances classified in Schedules I through V.

A closer look at the various sections of federal law pertaining to opioid prescribing should help clinicians to better understand the expectations of federal regulators and enforcement agents. Of particular interest to practitioners who prescribe and administer opioids is Part 1306, which covers the rules for prescriptions.

Registration[4]

- Every person who manufactures, distributes, dispenses, imports, or exports CS must register with the Drug Enforcement Administration (DEA) and must maintain that registration. Each registrant receives a number that is valid for 3 years.
- An exception allows a nonregistered agent or employee of a registered practitioner to administer or dispense CS in the course of normal professional practice. This exemption includes nurse practitioners and physician assistants.[5]
- A practitioner employed by a hospital or other registered institution can prescribe by using the institutional registration.
- The registrant must sign all prescriptions and is responsible for compliance with the CSA. It is important to remember that state or local laws may limit the prescribing power of agents or employees.
- A separate registration is required for each place of business or professional practice.
- The premises are subject to inspection to ensure compliance with regulations.

Records and Reports of Registrants[6]

- All registrants must keep complete and accurate inventories of CS on hand for each location and must keep those records separate from other records. Any CS returned by a patient or intended as free samples should be included in those records.
- All registrants must provide secure storage for CS.
- A registrant is required to keep records of CS dispensed to patients but is not required to keep records of CS prescribed during lawful practice unless those agents are prescribed in the course of addiction maintenance or detoxification.

Rules of Schedule II prescriptions:[7]

As CII medications, opioids are subject to the following regulations for prescribing:

- Issued by written prescription only.
- Written in ink or indelible pencil or typewritten.

- May be faxed, but the original must be presented to the pharmacist before the drug is dispensed. (Exceptions exist allowing CII prescriptions to be faxed as the original. Examples include medications for intravenous administration for patients in a long-term care facility such as a nursing home, retirement or mental-care facility, and for patients in hospice care).
- Signed by the registrant, who must include his or her full name, address, and registration number.
- Dated and signed on the day issued.
- Include the drug name, dose, dosage formulations, quantity prescribed, and directions for use.
- Verbal prescriptions (which are accepted only in emergency) must be confirmed within 72 hours.
- Not refillable.
- Not restricted in quantity or date of prescription expiration (state rules may apply).

If a pharmacist is out of stock of a particular opioid, he or she may dispense a partial quantity as long as the balance is filled within 72 hours. If that does not occur, the balance of the prescription becomes void. Exceptions are provided for patients in long-term care and for the terminally ill.[8]

Emergency Prescribing

The federal government allows a practitioner to deliver a verbal prescription to a pharmacist to request the delivery of painkilling drugs in an emergency when there is no time for a written prescription. The drugs must be necessary for treatment with no feasible alternative being available. The quantity of the CS must be equal to the medication required during the emergency period only. The pharmacist must try to confirm the identity of the prescriber, so practitioners should expect a call-back. A written prescription that is provided in person or by mail must immediately follow the verbal request. Written on the face of the prescription should be the words "Authorization for Emergency Dispensing" and the date of the verbal order. If the prescription has not arrived (or was not postmarked) within 7 days after the drug was supplied for the emergency situation, the pharmacist must notify the DEA.[9]

Treating the Pain of Addicted Patients

Federal permission to relieve pain with opioids extends to patients with an active addiction to narcotic substances. This is an issue fraught with confusion for many healthcare professionals, and the applicable law must be read and interpreted with care and caution.

The rules for the treatment of addiction are very different from those for pain treatment. A practitioner must have a special license to run an opioid treatment program (OTP)[2] to maintain a patient who is receiving methadone for the treatment of addiction. Unless one holds an OTP license, using any CS to maintain an addicted individual is not approved as a legitimate medical need and is forbidden. An exception is provided if an addicted person must undergo detoxification or be maintained in a hospital setting before surgery or before receiving other medical treatment unrelated to addiction. Federal law also allows a practitioner to administer (not prescribe) daily medication to prevent withdrawal for no longer than 3 days while arrangements for treatment are made.[2]

To summarize the rule, a non-OTP–licensed practitioner may use CS to treat the pain of an addicted person but may not use the same substance to treat addiction. Therefore, when the concern is analgesia rather than addiction maintenance, practitioners are allowed to prescribe opioid analgesics to treat addicted patients in intractable pain, even long term. Such prescribing or administering of opioids must be medically appropriate and within the standards set by the medical community. To avoid misunderstanding and unwanted regulatory scrutiny, it is vital to note in the patient's medical record that chronic opioids are indicated for "analgesia." Ambiguous terms such as "opioid maintenance" should be avoided. As always, state laws may impose additional restrictions.

Another question that arises is the legality of treating pain in an addicted patient who is enrolled in an OTP. When approached with this question, an official from the DEA Office of Diversion Control affirmed the practice as follows:

> Pain specialists may treat a chronic-pain patient currently enrolled in a narcotic treatment program with narcotics. The Controlled Substances Act does not set standards of medical practice. It is the responsibility of individual practitioners to treat patients according to their professional judgment for a legitimate medical purpose in accordance with generally acceptable medical standards.[10]

Once again, it is important to keep complete and accurate records to document that a pain syndrome is being treated, not the disease of narcotic addiction.

The Role of the DEA

The DEA, which is a division of the US Department of Justice, tracks the flow of an opioid from the point of manufacture until its final delivery to the patient or "ultimate user." It also enforces all tenets of the CSA, including those related to lawful prescribing. When a practitioner deviates from lawful prescribing, the DEA may respond in 2 ways:

- By acting to suspend or revoke the prescriber's registration to prescribe CII medications.
- By moving to indict the prescriber for alleged criminal acts.

The idea of being investigated is frightening to doctors and other healthcare professionals, although the risk of that event is slight. However, the commitment of drug enforcers at all levels — federal, state, and local — to fighting the "war on drugs" must not be minimized. This is serious business. The most potent weapon for protecting one's practice is to keep meticulous records documenting the purposes and outcomes of opioid administration. Specific steps for accomplishing this task follow later in this chapter.

How a drug-related investigation occurs

DEA inspectors are authorized to enter and inspect hospitals, clinics, and other premises in which CS are routinely stored and dispensed by prescription or other means of administration.[11] This includes access to all records and inventories. Financial records are excepted unless the physician or other person in charge agrees to release them. Researchers may petition to protect the privacy of subjects participating in research projects. All agents of the DEA and the Federal Bureau of Investigation are authorized to seize property for purposes of controlled-substance law enforcement.

The DEA inspector must:

- Make his or her presence known to the person in charge.
- State his or her purpose.
- Present credentials.
- Present a written notice of inspection authority or obtain consent.
- Conduct inspections at "reasonable times and in a reasonable manner."

The requirement for written authority does not apply to an establishment applying for initial registration or to investigations launched under exceptional circumstances, such as a threat to health or safety. If investigators deem that enough evidence against a CS registrant exists, possible actions include:

- A letter of admonition.
- An informal hearing.
- Civil penalties.
- Voluntary surrender of registration for cause.
- Revocation of registration.
- Arrest.

If a hearing is not scheduled, one may be requested (or waived). The practitioner accused of noncompliance with CS law will have the chance to present his or her views either orally or in writing and to propose ways of achieving compliance regarding the alleged violations.

The "Chilling Effect:" Myth or Reality?

Since 1999, when a General Accounting Office report criticized DEA efforts in battling drug abuse, the DEA has been under pressure to respond. Recent prosecutions of physicians who prescribe high doses of opioids have spread fear and mistrust among pain specialists.

Several surveys have shown that the fear of being scrutinized by a regulatory or law-enforcement agency compels many physicians to prescribe fewer opioids. Many physicians are particularly reluctant to prescribe opioids for their pain patients who do not have cancer. This unwillingness (caused by regulatory concerns) to treat pain is known among prescribers of opioids as the "chilling effect."

The DEA refutes the chilling effect and claims that such worries are unsupported by the relatively small number of actions that the agency takes against physicians. To prove its point, the DEA posted pie charts on its Web site showing that the agency pursued sanctions against less than one-tenth of 1% of registered US physicians from 1999 through 2003. Of 963,385 registrants for the partial year 2003, the DEA conducted 557 investigations that resulted in 441 actions against registrants and 34 arrests.[12] A common complaint driving these actions was that the registrants knew or should have known that their patients were abusing drugs. Pain-management specialists protested that those numbers are skewed because only a few practitioners prescribe the bulk of opioids, particularly in the large quantities needed by opioid-tolerant chronic-pain patients. Furthermore, they claimed that even if the number of actual disciplinary actions or prosecutions is small, doctors who perceive that they are in danger will be unwilling to prescribe for patients in pain.

Continuing the conversation at the 6th International Conference on Pain and Chemical Dependency, DEA chief diversion officer Patricia Good said that investigators are not trying to play "gotcha" with pain prescribers. She asserted that:[13]

- The DEA is looking for the appropriate documentation of opioid prescribing in medical records.
- The DEA is looking for evidence that patients are being monitored and that prescriptions are not being automatically renewed.
- Doctors are not prosecuted for information in their patients' medical charts alone.

To further allay fears, the DEA joined with 21 major healthcare organizations to call for a balanced approach to keeping prescription drugs available for medical purposes while battling drug diversion.[14] The document contained the following principles that support the prescribing of opioids for analgesia:

- Undertreatment of pain is a serious problem.
- Effective pain management is an important aspect of quality medical care.
- Pain should be treated aggressively.
- For many patients, opioids are the most effective treatment.

Yet at times, the zeal of the DEA to stop the flood of misused medications has led to actions that confuse and dismay pain-management specialists. One such event occurred when the DEA abruptly withdrew support for a document that had been the result of cooperation between regulators and pain experts. Citing "legal misstatements," the DEA removed the document titled "Prescription Pain Medications: Frequently Asked Questions and Answers for Health Care Professionals and Law Enforcement Personnel" from its Web site. One of the DEA's objections threw into question the longstanding prescribing practice of writing multiple prescriptions on the same day with instructions to fill some of those scripts on later dates. The agency equated this practice to an "illegal refill" of CII medications. In comments published in the DEA *Federal Register* of November 16, 2004,[15] the agency further refuted certain principles outlined in the frequently asked questions document and stated the agency's position that:

- The number of patients in a practice who receive opioids, the number of tablets prescribed, and the duration of opioid therapy may indeed indicate diversion.
- Physicians must never dispense a medication knowing that it will be used nonmedically or resold.
- Physicians must exercise a "greater degree" of oversight to prevent diversion if they are aware that a patient has resold medication or is an addict.
- Physicians should take seriously concerns about a patient's drug abuse that are conveyed by family members and friends.

Some of this language confused pain-management practitioners even further about the risks they might face when prescribing opioids. They protested the newly interpreted prescribing restriction in particular and argued that the results would be prescriptions written for a greater quantity of drugs, thus providing more opportunity for diversion, or patients in stable condition required to make more frequent and expensive office visits. After taking comments from interested parties, the DEA reversed itself 2 years after having introduced the prescribing limits and proposed a rule that, if finalized, would allow future CII prescriptions to be written for up to a 90-day supply. To its credit, the agency proved willing to listen to experts in pain management.

To clarify its own position and to distance itself from any suggestion that it wants to dictate the practice of medicine, the DEA took several additional steps. It:

- Replaced the frequently asked questions section with the document titled "Policy Statement: Dispensing Controlled Substances for the Treatment of Pain"[16] to clarify physicians' responsibility to take "reasonable measures" to prevent drug diversion.
- Updated the DEA *Practitioner's Manual* to further clarify physician responsibilities, including security measures for safeguarding CS and the reporting of theft.[17]
- Listed public facts from "Cases Against Doctors" on its Web site.[18]

These incidents illustrate the ongoing struggle to reach an understanding between regulators and healthcare practitioners and offer hope that greater cooperation will become the norm. It is clear that communication lines must be kept open to achieve the common goal of patient health and well-being.

Communication is perhaps even more vital at the state level. State laws and enforcement policies vary widely and are driven by local politics, sociological factors, crime and accident statistics, and cultural attitudes toward drugs and pain.

State Law: Opioid Prescribing

States, not the US government, set the professional standards for medical and pharmacy practice. States also write and enforce their own laws governing opioid prescribing. In addition to those mandates, state agencies in charge of health care and professional licensing create additional rules that must be followed. Because healthcare professionals must comply with all pertinent laws and policies, having a thorough familiarity with the legal tenets of one's home state is imperative. A good place to start is with the Web site of the state agency that licenses healthcare professionals.

Most state systems incorporate some combination of the following mandates:

- A Controlled Substances Act for each state.
- Rules and regulations governing CS prescribing.
- A medical practice law.
- A medical board that regulates standards of care.
- A medical and pharmacy licensing agency.
- Intractable Pain Treatment Acts (in 12 states).
- Guidelines and position statements, issued by state agencies, that address medical practice, pain management, opioid prescribing, and other related issues.

State requirements for opioid prescribing are often more strict than federal law. For example, although the federal CSA does not limit the size or expiration of a CII prescription, several states do; they limit prescription quantities to a 30-day supply, for example, or mandate that the prescription be filled within a few days after issuance. Unfortunately, some state regulations contain confusing, outdated or restrictive language pertaining to pain and addiction medicine. This is due in part to the Uniform Controlled Substances Act (UCSA), a model drug law offered to states to serve as a guide for creating their own drug laws. The UCSA contains positive measures but fails to ensure the availability of drugs or to define addiction among other shortcomings. Lacking a definition of addiction, terms such as "habitual user" or "habitué" have even led, in the past, to the reporting of cancer patients to the state. Large-scale adoption of the UCSA guidelines helped usher in state laws with no specific recognition of the value of opioid treatment for intractable pain.

In addition, states crafted their own unique drugs laws, some of which incorporated inconsistent or medically incorrect references to pain patients or addicted people. Frequently, the neurobiologic disease of addiction is confused with the normal physiologic response of physical dependence. Such confusion brings the potential for the incorrect application of the label "addict." Worse, in opposition to federal law, some states even appear to prohibit using CS to treat pain if the patient in pain also suffers from addictive disease.

Ironically, several states instituted those barriers while trying to create an environment friendlier to pain management with the passage of Intractable Pain Treatment Acts (IPTAs). The paradox presented by these laws is that although they purport to improve access to good pain care by recognizing the legitimacy of opioids, many contain language that introduces extra hindrances or mischaracterizes important concepts of pain management. Sometimes the language in an IPTA conflicts with the state's controlled substance laws, causing further confusion. IPTAs are falling out of favor, and few have passed in recent years.

The Role of State Medical Boards

State medical boards set the standards for medical practice. Most medical board members are themselves physicians. If a medical board finds evidence of inadequate professional standards, malpractice, or incompetence involving opioid prescribing, it may impose some combination of the following sanctions:

- Monitor the prescribing habits of a physician for a set period.
- Require the completion of continuing medical education hours on appropriate prescribing.
- Require voluntary surrender of a DEA registration for a set period.
- Suspend a physician's medical license for a set period.
- Revoke a physician's medical license for a set period.
- Revoke a physician's medical license permanently after a serious violation.

The criteria under which a state medical board will launch a full investigation of the prescribing or dispensing practices of a physician or other license holder varies from state to state. Some boards report that they investigate 1 complaint, and others establish a pattern of inappropriate prescribing. Authorities in 1 state may emphasize the enforcement of laws to prevent abuse and diversion, and another state's leaders are happy to leave prescribing quantities and other pain-management decisions up to professional judgment. In a few states, high quantities of prescribed opioids will trigger scrutiny, but other states are more cognizant of the patient-care patterns that accompany treatment for chronic pain.

It is a positive sign that medical board members are demonstrating better knowledge of issues pertinent to addiction and pain management than in the past. A survey of state medical officers showed they were more likely in 1997 than in 1991:

- To correctly distinguish between addiction and physical dependence.
- To agree that opioids are underutilized to treat cancer pain.
- To be less skeptical about the appropriateness of prescribing long-term opioids for chronic nonmalignant pain.[19]

A report published in the *Journal of Pain and Symptom Management* argued that the risk of a physician's facing discipline from a medical board solely for "overprescribing" opioids is nearly nonexistent. Of 120 US physicians disciplined during a 9-month period for problematic opioid prescribing, most were cited for multiple violations:

- 43% prescribed opioids for themselves or for nonpatients.
- 12% prescribed for addiction without addressing the problem.
- 42% kept inadequate records.
- 19% prescribed opioids when opioids were not indicated.
- 13% showed other types of incompetence.
- 8% engaged in sexual activity with patients.[20]

However, some of the parameters of that study are unclear. For example, no definition for the term "overprescribing" was given, and the term "inadequate records," which applied to the actions of nearly half of the physicians disciplined, can have several interpretations.

Regardless, that study could be considered a positive step, because it continues the trend toward reexamining drug-prescribing policy with the goal of ensuring that it does not deter prescribers from providing pain control. The next section will explore a prime impetus behind this improvement: the revision of US medical board guidelines to reflect a greater acknowledgment of the medical value of opioids.

Better Guidelines for Pain Treatment: The Federation of State Medical Boards Model Policy

In 1998, a positive development in policies of pain management occurred. Heralding a new and optimistic phase of reinvention, the Federation of State Medical Boards (FSMB) issued the *Model Guidelines for the Use of Controlled Substances for the Treatment of Pain*[21] as a guide for state medical boards to rewrite their own policies related to opioid prescribing. Amended in 2004 and renamed the "Model Policy," that document encourages the provision of treatment for pain, including the use of medical opioids for nonmalignant pain, and seeks to alleviate physician fears of regulatory discipline. It also aims to bring about greater consistency in the states' approach to pain management and opioid prescribing. By 2004, 22 states had adopted policies using all or part of the Model Policy.

Among the provisions of the Model Policy are the following tenets:

• Pain management is integral to quality medical care.
• Opioid analgesics for all types of pain may be essential for relief.
• Inappropriate pain management includes nontreatment, undertreatment, overtreatment, and the continuation of ineffective treatment.
• Sound clinical judgment and clear documentation of pain must accompany all CS dispensing.
• Physicians are not to be penalized solely for prescribing opioids in the course of providing legitimate medical care.
• Quality of care is not to be judged exclusively on the quantity of medication or duration of treatment.
• Nonmedical opioid use poses a threat to individuals and society.
• Physicians should reduce the potential for drug abuse and diversion.

The policy also updates definitions for addiction, physical dependence, and tolerance and outlines 7 treatment guidelines for good medical practice in opioid prescribing. Those treatment guidelines are summarized later in the chapter under "Steps that Protect a Practice."

As amended, the Model Policy emphasizes the continuing prevalence of undertreated pain as a deviation from acceptable standards of care. The policy further highlights the clinician's responsibility to assess patients' pain and to adjust doses or treatment plans accordingly.

Barriers to Treatment in State Law

State laws, regulations, and guidelines have come a long way, thanks in large part to the influence of the FSMB Model Policy. However, problems still remain. Not only are many state requirements stricter than federal law, they still vary greatly among states. Some of these requirements are used to override medical decisions with government decree.

The Pain and Policy Studies Group (PPSG), which is headquartered at the University of Wisconsin in Madison, leads the field in research into the impact of state pain policy on medical care and opioid prescribing. Reports issued by the PPSG discovered language within state statutes and guidelines that could erect barriers to good pain management. The group found that several states:

• Perpetuate confusion among addiction, tolerance, and physical dependence.
• Characterize the medical use of opioids as a last resort.
• Suggest that the medical use of opioids exists outside professional practice.
• Limit prescribing according to the quantity of the drug needed or the duration of treatment.
• Limit the length of prescription validity.
• Require specialist evaluation before opioids are prescribed to treat pain.[22]

The PPSG assigned each state a grade from A to F that is based on the extent to which policies that were intended to battle abuse and diversion pose the potential to interfere with patient care. Provisions within policies were designated as "positive" or "negative" according to how conducive they are to good pain management in relation to the principle of balance. The results of the Report Card indicate that progress toward the creation of more enlightened state pain policies is being made. Between 2000 and 2006, 35 of 51 states changed their policies on pain management enough to earn a grade improvement. Furthermore:

- In 2000, 29% of states earned above a grade C.
- In 2003, 41% of states earned above a grade C.
- In 2006, 82% of states earned above a grade C.[23]

However, some states still retain negative policies that could impede pain care, such as insisting that clinicians exhaust all treatment options before prescribing opioids. That policy would leave unclear how many options must be tried or how to address pain-relief needs in an emergency. The requirement to consult with a pain-management specialist before administering opioids ignores the needs of patients who require immediate treatment and causes needless delay if the treating practitioner is knowledgeable about pain management. Some states still use inaccurate definitions that confuse the consumption of opioids for pain management with addiction. Physicians' fear of regulatory action still presents a significant impediment to their willingness to provide pain relief.

The Progress Report Card serves as an example of what the chronic pain field needs much more of: research that, as the PPSG notes, "is the result of a systematic policy analysis rather than a statement of a 'position.'" Although problems remain, the overall message is positive: State pain-management policies are changing for the better.

The Rise of Pain-Control Advocacy

Federal and state authorities should place the same significance on the danger of pain undertreatment as they place on the battle against drug abuse and diversion. That theory sounds logical. Yet a review of the actions of state medical boards against licensees reveals that undertreatment is a relatively rare complaint. This may be changing, and undertreatment is becoming a growing concern for medical boards.

Most complaints of undertreatment are brought by patients' families. In 1999, the Oregon Board of Medical Examiners disciplined a physician for failing to provide adequate pain treatment because a patient was in such torment after her pain medication was withdrawn that she ripped out her own breathing tube.[24] In another case, a California internist was found guilty of elder abuse for failing to treat the pain of an 85-year-old nursing-home patient who was dying of mesothelioma. His daughter, arguing that her father's pain was medicated too late and too little, spoke of buying earplugs for his roommate to block out her father's dying moans. The internist admitted to prescribing an oral solution that is available only in tablet form. The medical board also censured the physician's directive to administer the medication "as needed," saying that it was meant to be given on a regular schedule.[25]

Cases such as these took on the weight of moral imperative as pain-control advocates grew more vocal and presented evidence of undertreated pain as a widespread public health problem in America. Actions by policy makers indicated that at least part of the message was getting through. In 2003, Congress introduced several bills to encourage the wider availability of pain care and to foster research and education. The chief measure eventually evolved into the National Pain Care Policy Act of 2005,[26] which, if passed, would increase funding for pain-related research and create several regional pain research and treatment centers.

The attention to undertreated pain is overdue, but the irony for clinicians is clear: Those who feared sanctions associated with the prescribing of opioids could now face discipline for undermedicating a patient with a legitimate need for pain relief. The principle of balance dictates that efforts to right a wrong must not tip the scale too far in the opposite direction. For clinicians, the resolution lies in a logical and compassionate approach to both pain treatment and drug-abuse prevention.

Drug Diversion: Prevalence and Sources

The increase in the illegal diversion of prescription pain medication is a threat to public and personal health that must not be ignored by the medical establishment. It is, however, a criminal issue, and one that needs a legal remedy rather than a medical one. Tension between the medical worldview and the perspective of enforcers is inevitable. Many clinicians wonder where their chief responsibility lies.

The principle of balance articulated by the DEA and many other government sources also applies to healthcare practitioners. It is critical to keep opioid analgesics available for patients who need them. It is also necessary to take any and all steps to help block the flow of narcotic painkillers into the hands of nonmedical users, many of whom are young people and first-time abusers. This does not mean that clinicians must become junior police officers or that they will never be fooled by a patient seeking to divert opioids to the black market for sale. It does mean, however, that pain-control advocacy must not become one-sided by insisting that undertreated pain poses the only possible harm to patients, and that the damage wrought by the illegal sale and misuse of opioids is negligible or of no concern to clinicians.

In a survey of state medical officers, 47% said that diversion had worsened in the past 5 years.[19] Although the perception of harm from drug diversion is high, definitive data on that issue are lacking. Government sources frequently speculate about both the prevalence and sources of diverted pharmaceuticals, because it is almost impossible to track a drug after it has been diverted, and it is difficult to distinguish between diversion and legitimate use. For example, the DEA reports that law-enforcement officials have been monitoring oxycodone products for abuse and diversion for 3 decades. However, exact statistics regarding drug diversion remain unclear. The best data have been obtained from localities: For instance, a survey of 34 law-enforcement agencies reported 5802 cases of diversion in the year 2000 alone.[27] Clearly, the problem of drug diversion is significant in the United States.

The uncertainty surrounding diversion statistics extends to knowing exactly where the diverted drugs are obtained. Judging from an amalgamation of reports,[28-30] the top sources of diverted pharmaceuticals in the United States are:

- Employees who steal from inventory.
- Prescription forgery.
- Robberies from pharmacies and drug distributors.
- "Doctor shoppers" (patients who seek pharmaceutical drugs from more than 1 provider).

- Pharmacists and pharmacy technicians who steal stock and falsify records.
- Physicians who sell prescriptions to drug dealers and abusers.
- Illegal Internet pharmacies.
- Illegal trafficking from Mexico and other foreign countries.

According to the DEA, most diverted pharmaceuticals result from illegal acts by physicians and pharmacists.[30] However, no exact statistics or other support for that pronouncement have been provided. Other evidence suggests that many drugs are smuggled into the country; US law-enforcement authorities are reporting an increase in the illegal trafficking of pharmaceuticals from Mexico and through Internet pharmacies.[30]

Given the frequent vagueness of official reports, the research completed by Joranson and Gilson, who analyzed data from 22 states by means of DEA records obtained through the Freedom of Information Act, is significant.[31] Their data show that a high degree of diversion occurs within the chain of pharmacy supply, either as theft from pharmacies or in the manufacturing and distributing of pharmaceuticals. Data from 2000 to 2003 showed that:

- Almost 28 million dosage units of controlled substances were diverted in 12,894 separate incidents that primarily involved theft and loss from pharmacies before the drugs were prescribed.

Six opioids were among the controlled substances diverted as shown in the following units:

- Oxycodone: 4,434,731.
- Morphine: 1,026,184.
- Methadone: 454,503.
- Hydromorphone: 325,921.
- Meperidine: 132,950.
- Fentanyl: 81,371.

The family medicine cabinet is a top source of diverted pharmaceuticals that is often ignored or minimized. According to a federal survey, adults who abused pain relievers nonmedically within the 12 prior months reported that they obtained the drugs as follows:

- 59.8% from a friend or relative for free.
- 16.8% from 1 doctor.
- 4.3% from a drug dealer or other stranger.
- 0.8% from the Internet.[32]

Anecdotal evidence suggests that many young people obtain products to sell or abuse directly from leftover or current supplies belonging to other family members. This is supported in a report that described "pharming parties" as a favorite social pastime of youthful abusers.[33] Those parties serve as venues for swapping handfuls of pills for preferred varieties. Because drug abusers steal medications belonging to others, clinicians should counsel patients to keep tight control of all prescriptions and to dispose of unused medications.

The Internet: The Electronic Pusher

The Internet is the latest lucrative market for illegal prescription-drug sales. Speaking at the 2007 annual meeting of the American Academy of Pain Medicine, drug diversion investigator John Burke characterized illegal Internet sales as "a huge issue" that involved the sale of millions of units.[34] Invitations like the examples in Box VII:2 pack e-mail in-boxes every day.

A study by the National Center on Addiction and Substance Abuse at Columbia University in New York found that 90% of 157 sites selling controlled drugs on the Internet did not require a prescription.[35] Calling the purchase of Internet pharmaceuticals "easy as candy," the Center offered the following additional findings:

- 41% stated that no prescription was needed.
- 49% offered "online consultation."
- 4% required that a prescription be faxed.
- 2% required that a prescription be mailed.
- 4% made no mention of prescriptions.

The DEA, which has been tracking online pharmacies, reports that it has found only 14 online pharmacies that fill prescriptions with proper clearance from physicians who have examined patients. The lack of physician clearance makes counterfeited and contaminated drugs an additional danger.

The *Star-Ledger*, a New Jersey-based newspaper, conducted its own investigation into the ease with which Internet drugs can be obtained. Of 6 controlled drugs ordered online, only a request for morphine was denied. The other 5 drugs purchased (oxycodone, hydrocodone, codeine, diazepam, and phentermine) were sent to a rented mailbox. Some medications arrived with prescriptions that were purportedly written by a physician. No medical consultation was required; only the submission of a completed online questionnaire was necessary to obtain the drugs.[36]

Researchers at the University of Pennsylvania School of Medicine in Philadelphia typed the words "no prescription codeine" into a search engine and found that of the first 100 commercial sites generated, 53 offered to sell medication without a prescription and many required only a payment method and a shipping address. Thirty-five of those sites also offered barbiturates, benzodiazepines, stimulants, and "date rape" drugs such as flunitrazepam and gamma hydroxybutyrate. About half the Internet sites were registered outside the United States, and 1 boasted a "less than one percent chance of your package being seized," citing the high volume of mail-order narcotics. Another site offered to reship for free if the package were confiscated.

The US Congress is attempting to address this easy access to drugs by introducing bills that set requirements for operating an Internet pharmacy and that mandate the disclosure of business information, such as the associated physician and pharmacist and the state of operation. Expanded enforcement powers would allow state authorities to take action in federal court to close Internet pharmacies.

In 2004, the White House also announced plans to find and prosecute unlawful Internet pharmacies via the use of new Web-based technologies. The FDA and DEA are making some progress in closing illegal Internet pharmacy sites; however, jurisdictional issues remain for Internet sites that originate in other countries.

Prescription Forgery

Forgery occurs in several ways. A diverter may steal a blank prescription and fill in the information or alter an existing prescription. A common trick is to alter the dosage quantity — for example, adding a zero to a "10," thus changing the number of doses prescribed to "100." Sometimes, the quantity of a drug prescribed is obscured with an opaque correction fluid and is then listed by the forger as a different quantity. Existing prescriptions may be rinsed blank with acetone such as that found in nail-polish remover and rewritten. Diverters may steal prescription pads or scan a prescription to make copies. Some forgers can create convincing prescriptions via the computer. A physician's signature can be scanned and printed with an ink cartridge printer. The resulting smudged signature may appear authentic to a pharmacist.

The telephone is also a leading drug-diversion tool. The diverter may alter the phone number written on a prescription and engage an accomplice to answer any calls for verification. A drug diverter may call in a prescription and provide his or her own telephone number for the pharmacist to call to confirm the validity of that prescription.

The Pain Connection

The extent to which the medical prescribing and administering of opioids for pain contributes to the availability of opioids for recreational abuse is a sensitive subject. Any attempt

---

Box VII:2   **Drugs on the Internet:***

We've assembled over 125 FDA-approved online pharmacies to deliver your hard-to-find brand and generic prescription drugs in one safe, secure, and discreet location without a prescription. Try our trial membership today.

Obtain All Meds A-Z with NO PRESCRIPTION

Buy OxyContin, Vicodin, Xanax, Valium, hydrocodone, Ritalin, Viagra, steroids, and more.
     Wholesale buyers welcome.

• No prior prescription required.
• Free medical consult.
• Easy online ordering.
• Only established and trusted pharmacies.
• FedEx delivery and worldwide shipping available.

* We have collected examples of statements found on Web sites and in online ads devoted to selling unauthorized pharmaceuticals. The Drug Enforcement Administration Office of Diversion Control invites concerned physicians and citizens to report suspicious Internet pharmacies.

to address this issue is subject to vocal protestations by pain-control advocates, who resist what they interpret to be any move to curtail the availability of opioids necessary for good pain management. The discussion of the issue is also subject to overzealousness by law-enforcement agencies that seek to control the supply of abusable narcotics and may label as a "pill mill" any establishment that provides opioids. Those who have that viewpoint fail to accept that undertreated pain is, like drug abuse, a bane of modern life.

Early evidence did suggest that the quantity of prescribing was not a major contributor to the rising tide of prescription-drug abuse.[37] However, because the percentage of opioids abused rose from 5.75% in 1997 to 9.85% in 2002, the same researchers conducted a new analysis and found that an increase in the quantity of opioids prescribed to treat pain has indeed coincided with an increase in the recreational abuse of those medications:

> "In our previous study ... data for 1990 to 1996 showed steadily increasing medical use and relatively low and stable levels of abuse ... At that time, we concluded that increased medical use of opioid analgesics did not appear to contribute to increased adverse health consequences. . . It is evident that in recent years increased medical use of several opioid analgesics is associated with increased abuse ..."[38]

This information does not negate the value of pain management. It only means that a greater ability to treat pain brings the unwanted effect of increased availability for drug abuse. As the researchers noted, "Intentional misuse of prescription controlled substances should not be allowed to compromise patient access to needed medications."[38] Once again, balance is the appropriate philosophy to apply to that dilemma.

The Battle Against Diversion

For professional diverters, prescription drugs offer advantages over street drugs. The strength and safety of the formulations in prescription drugs are guaranteed, oral use brings the user no risk of acquiring infection with the human immunodeficiency virus or hepatitis, and insurance or state benefits will sometimes cover all or part of the cost of purchase. Opioid analgesics, anxiolytics, anabolic steroids, and other CS have a high street value, and the lure of black-market profits is strong where economic distress dominates.

Signs of a Diverter

Pain-and-addiction lecturer Steven Passik, PhD, tells a story to illustrate how tough it is to ascertain whether a patient is diverting his or her medication. The patient in the story is a 70-year-old cancer survivor (not the typical profile for a diverter). Passik, a psychologist and palliative care specialist, joked self-deprecatingly that as a highly intuitive "student of human behavior," he knew that this patient was diverting his prescribed drugs "when the police brought him in wearing handcuffs."

Detecting a diverter is difficult at best. A drug diverter may be a patient, a coworker, a friend, or a relative. Some diverters have even masqueraded as government officials or pharmaceutical representatives.[39-40] Those traits are consistent from one practice to the next, and they are useful markers that clinicians can use to identify diverters. However, as any "student of human behavior" knows, the strict categorization of diverters is impossible.

It is evident that many of the behaviors on the list could also stem from logical and legitimate behaviors common to patients as well as diverters. For example, a patient may not show for a follow-up visit because he or she did not like the provider; patients who suffer chronic pain are frequently knowledgeable about pain medication names and strengths; or the patient may indeed be allergic to a specific substance in a prescribed drug, etc.

Although no behavior reliably indicates drug diversion, the chance of detecting such deception increases when clinicians watch for a pattern of behavior in their patients — for example, a patient who often psychologically pressures his or her physician for additional prescriptions by displaying an urgent need for those drugs. If a patient always demands immediate attention, is rushing to catch a plane or shows up unannounced near closing time to request a prescription, he or she may be seeking opioids for a nonmedical use. Such patterns indicate that something is wrong.

Diverters may be "street smart." They may be down on their luck and dress the part. But just as often, a diverter is a professional operator who is well dressed and articulate and is a model patient. It appears contradictory to warn clinicians that a patient may appear either overly knowledgeable or purposefully naïve in discussing medications, but the point is that such a patient is focused more on playing a role than on getting answers to address his or her medical condition.

Diverters may feign a pain syndrome and even fabricate symptoms. They have been known to prick a finger to put blood in urine or to wear a cast that suggests a nonexistent injury. Some diverters complain of pain that cannot easily be verified or discounted, such as abdominal or back pain, migraine, renal colic, toothache, or tic douloureux. Such deceptions are challenging for healthcare professionals who feel an ethical and professional obligation to believe a patient's claims of pain, which is a subjective experience.

The discussion thus far has centered on professional diverters, who exhibit no real medical condition and are seeking drugs to sell. Diverters may also be drug abusers who seek pharmaceuticals to sell to finance the purchase of their illegal drugs of choice. For that reason, it is important to check for signs of drug abuse such as new or old needle-track marks on the neck, axilla, forearm, wrist, foot, or ankle. Rarely, a diverter may be a patient in pain. A patient with few financial resources may sell extra pills to cover uninsured or underinsured costs to treat a legitimate pain problem.

When Confronted with a Suspected Diverter

Clinicians are often unsure about their responsibility when confronted with a suspected drug diverter. The DEA states that a healthcare professional is responsible for protecting his or her practice from becoming an easy target for diversion. In learning the potential dangers and safeguards, practitioners help uphold the law and protect society from drug abuse. It should be noted that federal law does not require a physician or other practitioner to contact law-enforcement authorities with information about an individual who has committed a crime. However, clinicians should be aware that criminal behavior is not bound by confidentiality, and a clinician violates no patient privacy laws if he or she does report such behavior.

The DEA outlines some specific guidelines that clinicians can use to block a would-be diverter:[40]

Box VII:3

Common Traits of Professional Diverters

- Refuses or is reluctant to present identification.
- Is "from out of town."
- Pays cash.
- Requests controlled substances by telephone.
- Schedules clinic visits for when the regular physician is unavailable.
- Is in a hurry.
- Requests drugs by name.
- Tries to control the interview.
- Is well versed in clinical or street terminology.
- Claims an allergy to nonsteroidal anti-inflammatory drugs, local anesthetics, or codeine.
- Gives reasons why alternative pain treatments will not work.
- Gives evasive answers.
- Does not show up for follow-up visits.
- Shows no interest in a diagnosis.
- Claims no health insurance.
- Has no regular physician.
- Claims that previous medical records are unavailable.
- Refuses physical examination.
- Attempts to skip diagnostic tests.
- Fakes naivete about medications or medical condition.
- Exaggerates or feigns symptoms.
- Feigns psychiatric symptoms of anxiety, insomnia, or depression.

- Perform a thorough physical examination and document the results.
- Document the questions asked of the patient and his or her responses.
- Request identification and a social security number. Photocopy these documents and include them in the patient's record.
- Call a previous practitioner, pharmacist, or hospital to confirm the patient's story.
- Confirm a telephone number at which the patient can be contacted.
- During each visit, confirm the patient's current address.
- Write prescriptions for limited quantities of drugs and do not postdate prescriptions.

Here are additional suggestions:

- Look for inconsistencies in the patient's medical history and take all possible action to verify the current complaint of pain.
- If you limit the quantity of drugs prescribed, ask the patient to schedule a follow-up visit.
- Train staff to respond to suspicious phone calls.
- Limit refills by phone and limit the number of staff members allowed to authorize refills. This policy will affect prescriptions for benzodiazepines and other non-CII medications.

• Never telephone prescriptions for an unfamiliar patient; insist that the patient make an appointment to come in.

It is important to trust one's instincts. Take precautions when you are suspicious, and never prescribe drugs simply to get rid of a drug-seeking patient. Ensure that all prescribing, dispensing, and administering of opioids and other CS are conducted within the scope of professional practice and as part of a practitioner-patient relationship.

Keep Prescriptions Secure

Measures to prevent illegal activities should be part of daily practice. Protecting access to prescriptions is a chief component.

• Never leave prescription pads where patients can access them.
• Never sign a blank or incomplete prescription.
• Write the quantity and strength of drugs prescribed in both numbers and letters.
• Use tamper-resistant prescription pads that cannot be photocopied.
• Do not preprint a CS-registrant number on a prescription pad.

Prescription Monitoring Programs: Advantages and Limitations

The prescription monitoring program (PMP) is a prime tool for identifying sources of diversion. As of 2006, 27 states had some form of monitoring program to track controlled-substance prescribing and dispensing. The data collected by PMPs are used to assist regulatory and law-enforcement authorities in investigating and preventing illegal practices. In some states, healthcare practitioners also may access data to ensure that patients are not obtaining opioids from more than 1 provider. This allows clinicians to assist in preventing diversion and helps prevent harmful drug interactions. Care must be taken to ensure that prescription databases are used only for professional (and never for personal) purposes.

The US General Accounting Office has studied the positive and negative effects of state PMPs[41] and reports that they:

• Are an effective tool for fighting diversion.
• Offer quick information on the drugs most likely to be abused.
• Deter doctor shopping.
• Have helped reduce the availability of abused drugs in Kentucky, Nevada, and Utah.
• Increase drug diversion activities in surrounding states that have no PMP.
• May reduce the number of prescriptions written for some controlled medications.

Data from Kentucky support the effectiveness of PMPs. The Kentucky All Schedules Prescription Electronic Reporting system (KASPER), which was implemented in 1998, was receiving 460 requests for reports each business day by 2003, and practitioners accounted for 85% of those requests. The National Drug Intelligence Center reports that the Kentucky system reduced the average time required for the completion of a drug investigation from 156 to 16 days.

Although this evidence shows that PMPs can be useful for detecting drug misuse, healthcare professionals, pain-control advocates, and patients are wary of the potential of the PMP for official misuse. Physicians worry that they may be labeled an "overprescriber" after an evaluation performed by a medically uninformed reviewer. Patients fear the loss of their confidentiality and being stigmatized as drug abusers. All parties involved with pain control want to ensure that official scrutiny does not result in clinicians' altering their prescribing practices, thereby reducing patient access to opioids needed for pain.

Evidence about whether PMPs diminish the willingness of clinicians to prescribe is contradictory. The overall production and consumption of CS have increased even though more states are collecting data; however, individual states with a PMP have recorded some decrease in the amount of CS being prescribed.

State PMPs: New Technology Results in Better Solutions

Some of the "fear factor" attached to prescription monitoring comes from a timeworn system that transmitted multiple copies of prescriptions to law-enforcement and government agencies. Multiple Copy Prescription Programs (MCPPs), or "triplicate" prescription programs, were implemented in the United States as early as 1913. MCPPs typically required that state-issued prescription pads containing serial numbers be used by clinicians. One copy of the completed prescription was sent to the state. That procedure caused misgivings about government oversight of medication decisions.

A lesson in prescribing anxiety was learned in California, where evidence showed that triplicate prescriptions reduced the abuse of CII medications but increased the abuse of CIII drugs, such as hydrocodone combined with acetaminophen, instead. By encouraging clinicians to circumvent the more regulated drugs, patients often failed to get the optimal drug, and the abuse problem simply shifted to a different schedule. California lawmakers heeded the evidence, repealed the triplicate requirement, and established instead a secure paper-prescription system backed by a computerized monitoring system.

Today, more states are favoring computer technology and are repealing multiple-copy serialized forms and replacing them with electronic data transmission (EDT) systems. EDT systems offer the advantages of:

- Quick turnaround for information requests.
- Removal of the distrust attached to government-issued prescription forms.
- Eliminating the need to generate multiple copies.
- Making data easier to compile and analyze than with a paper-based system.

An EDT information system used in conjunction with secure tamper-resistant prescription forms is quickly becoming the preferred method to track controlled medications. Secure forms provide security features (eg, ink that changes color when exposed to heat, fluorescent fibers that cannot be reproduced by copiers, instant voiding mechanisms that appear when exposed to scanning devices or ink-washing chemicals, embedded watermarks that can be used to identify genuine documents) that prevent forgery. Issued by government-approved printers, these secure forms eliminate the need to apply to an enforcement agency to receive serialized forms.

National Prescription Monitoring

After several years of tweaking and 2 previous failures to pass, a proposal to create nationwide prescription monitoring was signed into law in August 2005. The National All Schedules Prescription Electronic Reporting Act (NASPER) is intended to provide for multimillion-dollar grants for all 50 states to start or update their own programs for prescription monitoring. The national law also requires states to share information in an attempt to stop the increase in lawbreaking that occurs in states adjacent to those with a PMP. According to the National Drug Intelligence Center, the NASPER system will help track:

- Patient prescription use.
- Prescribing patterns of medical practitioners.
- Prescription rates for and usage patterns of specific drugs.
- Prescription patterns in geographic locations.
- Prescription patterns for long-term users.

Pain-management practitioners scrutinized the progress of the bill and wanted to ensure that it would benefit diversion-prevention efforts without hindering pain care. The American Society of Anesthesiologists lauded the focus of the final bill on the physician-patient relationship; the American Medical Association also supported the passage of the bill, but several pain-related associations did not.

The impact of nationwide prescription monitoring on patient care is yet to be seen. The goal is a system that gives law-enforcement authorities and regulators access to the monitoring capability they need while exempting them from day-to-day prescribing decisions reserved for clinicians. Ensuring that prescribing information is available to clinicians could help them to make good medical decisions and enhance patient safety. However, drug enforcers whose job it is to prevent diversion should think twice before declaring a program successful on the mere evidence that fewer prescriptions for opioids are being written. Such a statistic may indicate diminished patient care rather than a triumph of law enforcement.

Doctor Prosecutions: The Clinician's Legal Responsibility

The clinician's primary concern is the health and well-being of the patient. Because drug abuse places public health at risk, clinicians should help prevent diversion in any way possible. Prudent monitoring and meticulous recordkeeping are every clinician's responsibilities. However, physicians and other healthcare professionals cannot control all patient behavior, nor can they always detect a diverter.

The number of government actions against CS registrants may be small, but clinicians who prescribe large quantities of opioids, because they provide long-term treatment for the patients who have the most challenging and complicated chronic pain, appear to risk a higher degree of scrutiny than that applied to the average healthcare professional. Other practitioners who refuse to treat this population or who skimp on opioids for their acute-pain patients often answer to no higher authority than their own consciences.

The question of clinician culpability found a focus in William Hurwitz, MD. The Virginia physician, who was convicted of drug trafficking and racketeering among other charges,[42] is perhaps the most prominent physician prosecuted by federal enforcers in connection with opioid prescribing. The case drove a further wedge into the gap that separates the pain-control community from drug enforcers; both sides saw in the Hurwitz case a symbol of their worst fears realized. Pain-control advocates viewed Dr. Hurwitz as a physician who practiced compassion and good medicine by prescribing legal medication to patients in pain. To enforcement authorities, he was viewed as a clinician who supplied excessive amounts of dangerous drugs to addicts and black marketers. One question raised by the Hurwitz case concerns acceptable legal standards. The issue was whether physicians accused of wrongdoing are being mistakenly charged in the criminal system rather than appropriately dealt with through civil and administrative processes. Criminal prosecutions under CS law, in general, must show that clinicians knowingly acted to cause harm. Yet civil standard-of-care issues, such as alleged inadequate documentation or falure to conduct physical exams, have been introduced as evidence in criminal cases. The question of how to differentiate substandard medical care from a criminal action remains.

Another controversy centers on the expert witnesses chosen to determine the credibility of complaints against a clinician. Experts offer conflicting opinions involving such medical "gray areas" as the appropriateness of opioid administration for nonmalignant pain, the physician's obligation in matters of documentation, and the assignment of responsibility when a patient deviates from medical instruction. Protesting such inconsistency, pain experts want guidelines requiring an expert witness to:

- Be a full-time physician.
- Be active in medical practice.
- Be involved directly in patient care.
- Be knowledgeable about pain management.

The American Medical Association states that physicians who prescribe medication for patients in pain should not be burdened with "excessive regulatory scrutiny, inappropriate disciplinary action, or criminal prosecution"[43] and has called for state medical societies and boards to develop guidelines to protect physicians who prescribe opioids properly. California has taken the lead in crafting guidelines for complaints brought to the state medical board. Two experts must substantiate complaints involving prescribed medication for pain, 1 must be certified in pain management, and the other must be a practitioner in the same field as that of the physician undergoing investigation. Both experts must have treated patients during a significant part of the past 12 months. Perhaps similar guidelines in other states could help establish who is qualified to provide expert testimony in a criminal trial.

Nationwide, however, many problems remain. One difficulty is a tendency in the justice system to consider opioid-prescribing clinicians accountable for the deaths of patients, even if those patients were abusing the drugs prescribed, mixing prescriptions with illegal drugs or alcohol, or died from diseases unrelated to drug use. Furthermore, the practice of compiling lists of a state's "highest-prescribing physicians" fails to reflect accurately who may be abusing prescribing privileges, because a small percentage of clinicians treat the most difficult pain patients. Similarly, lists such as "the 100 most-monitored medications" could inhibit clinicians' willingness to legitimately prescribe those drugs.

If these issues remain undefined, neither enforcers nor those accused of crimes will understand precisely when a crime has occurred. However, the number of federal, state, and local enforcement agencies that are permitted to launch investigations of medical practices is daunting. Even if an investigation uncovers no wrongdoing, it can cost millions of dollars in defense efforts and can effectively shut down a practice, ruin reputations, and end careers. In a welcome development, some enforcers whose job it is to stop drugs from being diverted for illegal sale or use recognize the potential harm to society of hindering the availability of narcotic painkillers for legitimate pain. In a communication in a 2005 issue of the *American Medical News*, a past president of the National Association of Attorneys General warned government officials against harming good patient care: "We should concentrate on drugs that are illegally on the streets and work backward from that to find out how they got illegally on the streets. It should not be the other way around – looking at clinicians."

Steps That Protect a Practice

When a clinician knows and practices the guidelines for good patient care and keeps appropriate documentation, he or she increases the likelihood of productive partnerships between drug regulators and medical practitioners. However, sometimes the very nature of a clinician's practice invites regulatory scrutiny: Just as a patient's tendency to abuse opioids can be categorized as high risk, moderate risk, or low risk, so can the scope and quantity of a given clinician's prescribing habits present more or fewer warning signals to an investigator or enforcer (Box VII:4). The higher risk the practice, the greater the need for strict adherence to the rules of prescribing.

It is crucial to keep detailed documentation to protect a practice in the event of an investigation or any allegation of deviant professional conduct. This careful recordkeeping is also the best way to provide optimal patient care. A general overview of sufficient documentation is contained in Box VII:5. In addition, physicians and other clinicians should never prescribe opioids for members of their own family or for friends unless the medical records of those individuals clearly document a clinician-patient relationship. In some localities, such prescribing is forbidden. The following section further explains the protective steps outlined by the Federation of State Medical Boards. Some of the information echoes the clinical requirements listed in the chapter on monitoring patients, this time with an emphasis on protecting the clinician's practice.

Model Policy Treatment Guidelines

An important principle of good prescribing contained in the Federation of State Medical Boards Model Policy says that the quality of care is not based solely on prescription size, quantity, or duration of treatment and suggests that the chief criterion by which to judge a clinician's choices is the treatment outcome. The policy outlines 7 specific guidelines for using CS to treat pain. To give healthcare professionals a clearer idea of what is required, we will examine each of these steps in greater detail:

1. *Evaluate the patient.* Gathering a medical history and conducting a thorough physical examination is one of the most important steps to document. Disciplinary actions often center on a real or perceived lack of sufficient physical evaluation of the patient. According to the Model Policy, the patient evaluation should contain:

- The type of pain and its intensity.
- All current treatments and those tried in the past.
- Underlying and coexisting diseases or conditions.
- An evaluation of the impact of the pain on physical and psychologic function.

- Whether a history of substance abuse exists.
- One or more recognized medical indications for the use of opioids.

The last item is vital. Medical examiners and regulators want the administration of opioids justified in the medical record. If a diagnosis of a painful condition exists, document it thoroughly and provide support from all diagnostic, laboratory, and imaging tests. Call former healthcare providers as necessary to gather supporting information. Be sure also to account for any adjunct medications given to manage depression, anxiety, insomnia, or other coexisting conditions.

2) *Establish a treatment plan and put it in writing.* The treatment plan should be updated periodically to include all changes in medication or dosage noted. Decide whether nonopioid modalities would benefit the patient and whether help from experts in a different specialty is needed.

After a treatment plan has been selected, state the goals to be met and the criteria for meeting them. Treatment goals should focus on providing adequate pain relief and improving the patient's physical and psychosocial function and quality of life. Listen carefully to the patient to identify the obligations and challenges that his or her lifestyle entails.

Box VII:4   High-risk, Moderate-risk and Low-risk Prescribing Practices

High Risk: This category contains the top 1% of physicians who prescribe the bulk of opioid analgesics. Some clinicians will put their own reputations and livelihoods on the line to treat the most difficult patients. Should the regulatory "red flags" that come with the territory of a practice devoted to chronic-pain treatment spell automatic trouble for such a practitioner? At times, such scrutiny comes not from enforcement authorities but from representatives of state-run insurance organizations who wish to influence physicians away from their "expensive" medical decision making. The result is another form of intimidation.

Moderate Risk: The average physician or other practitioner who prescribes opioids for pain in a practice that is not exclusively devoted to chronic pain is unlikely to attract trouble from the Drug Enforcement Administration or state medical board.

Low Risk: The clinicians at lowest risk for regulatory investigation may be placing patients at risk for needless suffering from untreated or undertreated pain. Some clinics feature signs on the reception desk declaring certain classes or trademarks of opioid medications to be unavailable, thus implying they are a virtual abomination. Several motivations may drive low-risk prescribing. The perception that a regulatory investigation could take place can discourage some clinicians from prescribing needed medications. Other clinicians falsely believe that all or most patients who receive long-term opioid therapy will eventually become addicted. Still others equate the ability to stoically suffer pain with strong character.

Which activities are most important to the patient? What would he or she most like to see restored in life? Acknowledge that not all pain can be completely relieved and set realistic, attainable short-term and long-term goals that are based on the patient's priorities.

If a clinical trial of opioids is selected, the drug prescribed should be compatible with the diagnosis and should be adjusted according to the individual needs of the patient. The patient's progress and any further diagnostic evaluations, surgeries, or other treatments should be documented.

3) *Obtain informed consent and agreement for treatment.* Any patient for whom CS is prescribed to relieve pain should be informed of the potential risks and benefits of that medication. It is good practice to discuss (after obtaining the patient's permission) the accepted treatment plan with the patient's family members or significant other(s). Ensuring that the patient's family members understand what to expect is important, because they are a frequent source of complaints to regulatory agencies about opioids prescribed for their loved ones.

The patient should be counseled about the importance of complying with all treatment instructions and should understand and agree to the consequences of deviating from medical direction. The patient should receive opioid analgesics from only 1 clinician and 1 designated pharmacy whenever possible. A policy on the use of urine or blood screenings to

---

Box VII:5   Information for Inclusion in the Patient's Medical Record

- A medical history, including all available prior physical findings.
- The results of a physical examination.
- Support for the diagnosis of a painful condition.
- Initial and ongoing justification for opioid treatment. In some states, this includes a requirement for documentation that alternative treatment methods were tried and failed. Even when no such mandate exists, it is good practice to record the type, duration, and outcome of all previous treatment modalities.
- Diagnostic, therapeutic, and laboratory results.
- Verification and content of all consultations with other clinicians (including mental-health, substance-abuse and pain-specialist professionals) or their evaluations of the patient.
- A treatment plan that lists the long-term and short-term goals of treatment.
- An informed consent and treatment agreement signed by the patient and the clinician.
- A record of medications, including the date, type, dosage, and quantity prescribed.
- All treatment changes, surgeries, dose adjustments, etc.
- Proof that the patient was evaluated at regular intervals.
- A record of instructions and counseling provided for the patient.
- A record of ongoing assessments of pain relief, physical function, quality of life, and aberrant drug-related behavior.
- Documented awareness of any history of substance abuse and the ways in which it was addressed. Clearly note that opioids were prescribed for the treatment of pain and not for addiction maintenance.

determine compliance should be set and discussed. The patient's responsibilities should be clearly delineated, and the circumstances in which drug therapy may be discontinued should be explained. The clinician should strongly consider the use of a written agreement outlining all these expectations. That document should be signed by the clinician and the patient, particularly when a patient has a history of substance abuse. Opioid treatment agreements are discussed in Chapter VI.

4) Perform a periodic review. It is not sufficient to make a monthly notation in a patient's chart to document that the medication regimen is satisfactory and the prescription will be renewed. The patient's medical record must include the results of regular appointments and ongoing assessments of treatment progress. Depending on the patient's response to opioid therapy, the clinician may maintain or change the treatment plan. The patient's medical record should reflect the state of his or her health. Note changes in pain intensity, adjustments to medication or other treatments, and important life-changing events such as surgery, an accident, or other stressors related to family life, social environment, and work. Record any aberrant drug-related behavior observed during opioid therapy and the methods used to address it. Include the results of urinalysis and other compliance screening.

Consider the patient's progress in terms of the Four A's outlined in Chapter VI:

• Analgesia.
• Activities of daily living.
• Adverse events.
• Aberrant drug-related behaviors.

The goal is to determine whether the chosen treatment modality is resulting in less pain and an improvement in physical function and quality of life. If the patient is not making progress or if adverse effects are unmanageable after a reasonable treatment interval during which sufficient medication adjustments have been tried, it may be appropriate to consider alternative pain therapies.

5) Consult with professional colleagues as needed. Refer patients to appropriate professionals in the fields of psychiatry, cognitive or behavioral therapy, physical rehabilitation, addiction treatment, or other specialties as needed. Be prepared to manage the patient's pain condition in tandem with comorbid psychiatric disorders, substance abuse, or other conditions. Patients with multiple disorders will likely need a heightened level of monitoring, documentation, and consultation.

6) Keep complete and accurate medical records. These should be kept current and available for review. See Box VII:5 for more detail.

7) Comply with CS law. Compliance with law includes all relevant federal, state, and local mandates. State medical boards and licensing agencies can provide practitioners with specific state requirements.

A briefer protocol of the steps to protect a prescriber of opioids from legal or regulatory action is provided in Box VII:6.

Discharging the Noncompliant Patient

If a patient has committed a criminal act such as diversion, the clinician must terminate medical treatment and discharge the patient from care. Some state laws may require the reporting of this activity to the authorities. In a case of opioid abuse, the clinician may continue pain treatment with intensified monitoring, patient counseling, and careful documentation of all directives and outcomes. If egregious, intractable, aberrant behavior continues in addition to the continued deterioration of the patient's pain condition, the decision may be made to discontinue opioid treatment. Patients may also be discharged from opioid therapy not for any wrongdoing but because that treatment has become ineffective or is contributing to a diminished quality of life.

When such actions become necessary, certain questions are raised:

- Is it a clinician's responsibility to taper opioid therapy if the treatment must be discontinued?
- Is it a clinician's responsibility to offer referrals if a patient must be discharged from the clinic practice?
- What impact, if any, does a signed agreement about opioid treatment have on issues of patient abandonment?

Practitioners can be sued for patient abandonment if medical care is discontinued without justification after a clinical relationship has been established. In general, harm to the patient must be proven for that patient to win such a case. The ethics manual of the American College of Physicians gives these directives for discontinuing the professional relationship "under exceptional circumstances:"

- Notify the patient of the termination of the physician-patient relationship.
- Try to find adequate care elsewhere for the patient.
- Guard the patient's health in the process.
- Transfer medical information to another healthcare provider.
- Ensure continuity of care to the greatest extent possible.[44]

> "Physician-initiated termination is a serious event, especially if the patient is acutely ill, and should be undertaken only after genuine attempts are made to understand and resolve differences."[44]

Little direction specifically geared to the termination of opioid-treated pain patients is available. Guidelines from the American Academy of Pain Medicine (AAPM), the American Pain Society (APS), and the American Society of Addiction Medicine (ASAM) offer no directives for the discontinuation of opioid treatment resulting from noncompliance. In the absence of specific guidelines, a clinician must try his or her best. To avoid patient abandonment, the clinician who terminates a patient's treatment must make a good-faith effort to refer that patient to another qualified healthcare provider. If opioid therapy must be dis-

Box VII:6	**Protocol to Protect an Opioid Prescriber***

1. Evaluate the patient as follows:
   - Medical history.
   - Physical examination.
   - Pain type and intensity.
   - Treatments tried.
   - Coexisting diseases and conditions.
   - Impact of pain on physical and psychologic function.
   - Substance abuse history.
   - One or more recognized medical indications for the use of opioids.

2. Establish a treatment plan:
   - Set goals and criteria.
   - Update the treatment plan periodically.
   - Document the patient's progress.

3. Obtain informed consent.
   - Explain the risks and benefits of the prescribed medication.
   - Counsel the patient about the importance of compliance.
   - Counsel the patient about the consequences of noncompliance.
   - Strongly consider asking the patient for a signed agreement about his or her treatment.

5. Consultation as needed in fields of:
   - Psychiatry.
   - Cognitive or behavioral therapy.
   - Physical rehabilitation.
   - Addiction treatment.
   - Other specialties.

   Manage pain in tandem with comorbid conditions.

6. Keep complete, accurate medical records as detailed in Box VII:5.

7. Comply with federal, state, and local controlled substances laws.

* Modified from the Federation of State Medical Boards of the United States. Model policy for the use of controlled substances for the treatment of pain. Available at: http://www.fsmb.org/pdf/2004_grpol_Controlled_Substances.pdf. Accessed April 10, 2007.

continued in an addicted patient, consultation with a specialist in addiction medicine is recommended.

The discharge process is facilitated if the clinician has previously obtained from the patient a signed document of informed consent and a signed treatment agreement that includes reasons for which drug therapy may be discontinued. If a patient violates the written contract, a practitioner is within his or her rights to terminate the contract. Indeed, to protect one's practice, it is necessary to follow through with enforcement of all written agreements. All due effort should be made to secure appropriate continuing medical attention. However, a clinician is under no obligation to continue to provide opioids to patients who display egregious aberrant behaviors and cannot be trusted. This is particularly true if there is a chance of the patient's harming himself or herself.

Forging Partnerships: Separate Functions, Common Goals

The days when leaders in medicine and law enforcement could afford the luxury of choosing sides or squaring off against each other to protect their turfs are over. "Cooperation" must be the new watchword if an enemy as complicated and insidious as drug abuse is to be bested. Perhaps the first step is for pain-management specialists and other clinicians to acknowledge the damage of prescription opioid abuse and to vow to be part of the solution to stop its spread. For their part, DEA investigators, pharmacists, and members of state regulatory agencies would do well to inform doctors of suspected problems with patients' opioid intake.

Unfortunately, tunnel vision afflicts every profession. Workers in 1 field often see only the necessity of performing their own function and miss the big picture. Greater understanding of the missions and motivations that drive other professionals is vital. Drug officials and clinicians should not be natural enemies but partners in keeping opioids away from those who would use them for a detrimental purpose. To accomplish common goals, communication between professions must improve, because professionals in different specialties may interpret the same event very differently. Certain "red flags" that could cause someone in law enforcement to suspect prescription misuse may appear to be perfectly legitimate practice to a pain-management specialist (Box VII:7). To determine the true motivation behind such indicators, it is worthwhile to attend the meetings, conferences, and seminars sponsored by members of an associated profession and also to create joint training programs to turn the tide of drug abuse and undertreated pain.

Drug enforcers should:

- Understand pain-management guidelines.
- Leave abuse and addiction treatment to clinicians.
- Fight criminal diversion of drugs.

Clinicians should:
- Manage pain.
- Treat abuse and addiction as medical conditions.
- Cooperate in fighting drug diversion.

Honest clinicians abhor the diversion of drugs to places where they are sold or consumed for no medical purpose, but training is sometimes lacking. Although all states require continuing medical education (CME) to keep medical licenses current, content pertaining to CS prescribing is often not provided. The DEA has announced plans to work with state medical boards to add such a training component on opioid use to CME requirements for all physicians.

Enlightened policies about pain add little quality to patient care if no one knows about them. Education on the principles of pain management and the medical benefits of opioid therapy should be provided to leaders in local law-enforcement agencies, where decisions may be ruled by a philosophy of pure enforcement. State medical boards and licensing agencies are prime candidates to take the lead in alerting physicians and other clinicians, regulators, law-enforcement authorities, patients, and the public about improved standards of care related to pain management and addiction control. Web sites, seminars, newsletters, radio, and television provide ways to get the word out. The updating of training manuals and other educational materials for investigators is fundamental.

The Pharmacist as Partner

An understanding of pharmacists' professional and ethical obligations would enable clinicians to better partner with them to prevent abuse and diversion. Like healthcare practitioners, pharmacists answer to federal and state authorities to ensure that all prescriptions they dispense are accurate and valid. Pharmacists and healthcare practitioners authorized to prescribe CS are bound by law in a partnership known as "corresponding responsibility." It is the pharmacist's duty to question the validity of prescriptions.

Therefore, it is also the pharmacist's legal responsibility to challenge any CII prescription that does not seem correct. Ink that doesn't match or an unfamiliar signature on a written prescription are good reasons for a pharmacist to double-check that prescription's validity. If an emergency prescription for an opioid is dispensed and the practitioner does not provide the requisite written prescription within 7 days, the pharmacist must report the lapse to the DEA or risk facing government penalties.

It is important to remember that the pharmacist does not have access to a patient's medical record and may lack specific knowledge about pain management. A study of attitudes among Wisconsin pharmacists revealed that many considered the dispensing of opioids for more than a few months to patients with chronic pain to be unlawful.[45] Be ready to answer questions and to reassure the pharmacist of acceptable medical practice standards. The dispensing of prescriptions written for large quantities of drugs can be facilitated by a quick phone call from the prescriber to the pharmacist. It helps to indicate "chronic-pain patient" in writing on the prescription itself. It is also good practice to provide the pharmacist with copies of opioid agreements signed by the patient and physician.

If a clinician suspects a problem with diversion, it is a good idea to discuss this with the pharmacist and with other providers in case the patient has been "shopping." Practitioners and pharmacists concerned about privacy laws should know that it is legal under the Health Insurance Portability and Accountability Act (HIPAA) to speak with another healthcare professional about a patient as long as both are doing so from concern for the patient's care.

Box VII:7

"Red Flags:" Same Behavior, Different Perception

1) The patient travels a long distance to get opioids.
   The regulator sees: A "doctor shopper" or determined abuser.
   The clinician sees: A pain patient seeking expertise unavailable in his or her home-town.

2) The practitioner prescribes large quantities of opioids.
   The regulator sees: A dispenser of painkillers to serve no legitimate medical purpose.
   The clinician sees: A compassionate caretaker committed to treating long-term in-tractable pain.

3) The dose prescribed is potentially lethal.
   The regulator sees: Incompetence that could kill an opioid-naïve patient.
   The clinician sees: A commitment to treating opioid-tolerant patients who need high doses of medication to achieve analgesia.

4) The patient asks for drugs by name.
   The regulator sees: A "drug seeker" who may want to divert medications for sale.
   The clinician sees: An experienced pain-management patient who knows which drugs relieve his or her pain.

5) The patient returns too early for an office visit.
   The regulator sees: A medication misuser or diverter seeking more pills.
   The clinician sees: A patient whose pain has worsened and who requires immediate treatment.

6) The practitioner directs the patient to use multiple pharmacies.
   The regulator sees: A "doctor shopper."
   The clinician sees: A frightened pharmacist who will not dispense large quantities of a particular drug. The patient must then have prescriptions filled at several pharma-cies.

7) Multiple types of drugs are prescribed.
   The regulator sees: Drug diversion.
   The clinician sees: The pharmacologic remedies for comorbid conditions such as pain, anxiety, depression, or insomnia.

Adapted from Brushwood DB. Drug control policy out of balance. Pain & The Law. Available at: http://www.painandthelaw.org/mayday/brushwood_090403.php. Accessed April 2, 2007.

Conclusion

In an interview with the magazine *Pain Matters,* L. Jean Dunegan, MD, highlighted the need to eschew black-and-white thinking to find realistic solutions.[46] "In a perfect world, we could catch everyone engaging in illegal drug dealing and diversion, successfully rehabili-tate every drug abuser, fully treat every pain patient to the maximum of existing technology, and yet leave the freedom of everyone else uncompromised. We do not live in such a world."

It has been said that government provides the difficulty for every solution. It is true that despite good intentions, official efforts against diversion sometimes clash with clinicians' goals of providing patients with adequate pain control. However, it is also true that the government's goal of preventing abuse and diversion of CS is worthy.

To provide optimal patient care and to protect against unwanted regulatory scrutiny, a clinician should be familiar with all state and federal laws, use prescription monitoring if available, and document all aspects of opioid therapy.

Ultimately, government regulators and law-enforcement authorities must trust the healthcare community to use good medical judgment to treat pain. Governments cannot practice medicine; neither can healthcare practitioners serve as drug enforcers. Only through cooperation are both jobs performed successfully.

Using the Guidelines: Online Resources

The following online organizations present prescribing guidelines and safeguards for protecting a medical practice.
- Joint Commission on the Accreditation of Healthcare Organizations: www.jcaho.org.
- American Pain Society: www.ampainsoc.org.
- American Academy of Pain Medicine: www.painmed.org.
- National Cancer Care Network: www.nccn.org.
- World Health Organization: www.who.int.
- Federation of State Medical Boards of the United States: www.fsmb.org.
- Pain and Policy Studies Group, University of Wisconsin: www.medsch.wisc.edu/painpolicy.
- The Drug Enforcement Administration Web site for the Office of Diversion Control offers a summary of prescribing law (Code of Federal Regulations and codified Controlled Substances Act), Federal Register Notices and much more: http://www.deadiversion.usdoj.gov.
- An electronic version of the Code of Federal Regulations (e-CFR) is kept current online at the Web site of the US Government Printing office: http://www.gpoaccess.gov

---

References

1. Fitzhenry RI, ed. *The Harper Book of Quotations*. 3rd ed. New York, NY: HarperCollins; 1993:185.
2. Code of Federal Regulations, Title 21 CFR §1306 Prescriptions §1306.07.
3. Code of Federal Regulations, Title 21 CFR §1306 Prescriptions §1306.04.
4. Code of Federal Regulations, Title 21 CFR §1301 Registration of Manufacturers, Distributors, and Dispensers of Controlled Substances.
5. Code of Federal Regulations, Title 21 CFR §1301 Registration of Manufacturers, Distributors, and Dispensers of Controlled Substances §1301.22.
6. Code of Federal Regulations, Title 21 CFR §1304 Records and Reports of Registrants.

7. Code of Federal Regulations, Title 21 CFR §1306 Prescriptions.

8. Code of Federal Regulations, Title 21 CFR §1306 Prescriptions §1306.13.

9. Code of Federal Regulations, Title 21 CFR §1306 Prescriptions §1306.11.

10. Good P. DEA: Pain management in addiction medicine. Drug Enforcement Administration, US Department of Justice; March 2000.

11. Code of Federal Regulations, Title 21 CFR §1316 Administrative Functions, Practices, and Procedures §1316, Subpart A.

12. The myth of the "chilling effect: Doctors operating within bounds of accepted medical practice have nothing to fear from DEA [news release]. Washington, DC: DEA, US Department of Justice; Oct. 30, 2003. www.usdoj.gov/dea/pubs/pressrel/pr103003p.html. Accessed Nov. 9, 2005.

13. Good P. Regulatory issues. The 6th International Conference on Pain and Chemical Dependency. Brooklyn, NY; February 4-7, 2004.

14. Drug Enforcement Administration. A joint statement from 21 health organizations and the Drug Enforcement Administration. Promoting pain relief and preventing abuse of pain medications: a critical balancing act. J Pain Symptom Manage. 2002 Aug;24(2):147.

15. Interim policy statement: dispensing of controlled substances for the treatment of pain. Fed Regist. 2004:69(220):67170-67172.

16. Policy statement: dispensing controlled substances for the treatment of pain. Fed Regist. 2006; 71(172): 52715-52723. To be codified at 21 CFR § 1306.

17. Practitioner's manual: an informational outline of the controlled substances act. 2006 ed. DEA Office of Diversion Control Web site. Available at: http://www.deadiversion.usdoj.gov/pubs/manuals/pract/index.html. Accessed April 10, 2007.

18. Cases against doctors.. DEA Office of Diversion Control Web site. Available at: http://www.deadiversion.usdoj.gov/crim_admin_actions/index.html. Accessed April 10, 2007.

19. Hoffmann DE, Tarzian AJ. Achieving the right balance in oversight of physician opioid prescribing for pain: the role of state medical boards. J Law Med Ethics. 2003 Spring;31(1):21-40.

20. Richard J, Reidenberg MM. The risk of disciplinary action by state medical boards against physicians prescribing opioids. J Pain Symptom Manage. 2005 Feb;29(2):206-12.

21. Federation of State Medical Boards of the United States. Model policy for the use of controlled substances for the treatment of pain. Available at: http://www.fsmb.org/pdf/2004_grpol_Controlled_Substances.pdf. Accessed April 10, 2007.

22. Pain and Policy Studies Group. Achieving balance in federal and state pain policy: a guide to evaluation. 3rd ed. University of Wisconsin Paul P. Carbone Comprehensive Cancer Center. Madison, Wisconsin; 2006.

23. Pain and Policy Studies Group. Achieving balance in state pain policy: a progress report card. 2nd ed. University of Wisconsin Paul P. Carbone Comprehensive Cancer Center. Madison, Wisconsin; 2006.

24. Dembner A. Failure to treat pain target of lawsuits. The Boston Globe. 2003; November 8.

25. Kleffman S. Clinician disciplined over pain treatment. Contra Costa Times. 2004; January 17.

26. Office of Legislative Policy and Analysis. Bill tracking: H.R.1020—The National Pain Care Policy Act of 2005. Available at: http://olpa.od.nih.gov/tracking/109/house_bills/session1/hr-1020.asp. Accessed April 10, 2007.

27. Inciardi J, Goode J. OxyContin and prescription drug abuse: miracle medicine or problem drug? Consumers Research Magazine. 2003;86(July).

28. Zacny J, Bigelow G, Compton P, Foley K, Iguchi M, Sannerud C. College on Problems of Drug Dependence taskforce on prescription opioid non-medical use and abuse: position statement. Drug Alcohol Depend 2003 Apr 1;69(3):215-32.

29. Kraman P. Drug abuse in America — prescription drug diversion. TrendsAlert: Critical information for state decision-makers. The Council of State Governments. Available at: http://www.csg.org. Accessed April 4, 2004.

30. Drug Enforcement Administration, US Department of Justice. OxyContin: Pharmaceutical Diversion, Drug Intelligence Brief, March 2002. Available at: http://www.avitarinc.com/pdf/Drug-Intelligence-Brief-Oxycotine-Facts.pdf. Accessed April 10, 2007.

31. Joranson DE, Gilson AM. Drug crime is a source of abused pain medications in the United States. J Pain Symptom Manage. 2005 Oct;30(4):299-301.

32. Substance Abuse and Mental Health Services Administration. (2006). Results from the 2005 National Survey on Drug Use and Health: National Findings (Office of Applied Studies, NSDUH Series H-30, DHHS Publication No. SMA 06-4194). Rockville, MD.

33. Banta C. Trading for a high. Time Magazine. 2005; August 1:35.

34. Burke J. Drug diversion versus pain management: finding a balance. The 23rd annual meeting of the American Academy of Pain Medicine. New Orleans, LA; February 7-10, 2007.

35. "You've Got Drugs!" Prescription Drug Pushers on the Internet. National Center on Addiction and Substance Abuse (CASA) at Columbia University, New York, NY; February 2004.

36. Orr JS. Of six bogus requests for drugs over the Internet, only one was denied." Newark Star-Ledger; November 30, 2003.

37. Joranson DE, Ryan KM, Gilson AM, Dahl JL. Trends in medical use and abuse of opioid analgesics. JAMA. 2000 Apr 5;283(13):1710-4.

38. Gilson AM, Ryan KM, Joranson DE, Dahl JL. A reassessment of trends in the medical use and abuse of opioid analgesics and implications for diversion control: 1997-2002. J Pain Symptom Manage. 2004 Aug;28(2):176-88.

39. Cole BE. Recognizing and preventing medical diversion. Fam Pract Manag 2001 Oct;8(9):37-41.

40. DEA Office of Diversion Control, US Department of Justice. Don't be scammed by a drug abuser. Published 1999:1(1). Available at: http://www.deadiversion.usdoj.gov/pubs/brochures/drugabuser.htm. Accessed April 10, 2007.

41. US General Accounting Office (GAO). Prescription drugs: state monitoring programs provide useful tool to reduce diversion, May 2002. Washington, DC: GAO publication No. GAO-02-634.

42. Markon J. Pain doctor convicted of drug charges: Va man faces possible life term on trafficking counts. Washington Post. December 16, 2004.

43. American Medical Association. About the AMA position on pain management using opioid analgesics, 2004. Available at: http://www.ama-assn.org/ama/pub/category/11541.html, accessed March 1, 2004.
44. Ethics manual. Fourth edition. American College of Physicians. Ann Intern Med 1998 Apr 1;128(7):569-71.
45. Joranson DE, Gilson AM. Pharmacists' knowledge of and attitudes toward opioid pain medications in relation to federal and state policies. J Am Pharm Assoc (Wash). 2001 Mar-Apr;41(2):213-20.
46. The national voluntary monitoring system of controlled substance prescribers. Pain Matters: Partners Against Pain Magazine. Stamford, CT. Available at: http://www.partnersagainstpain.com/PainMatters/article3.asp. Accessed April 10, 2007.

CHAPTER VIII

EMERGING RESEARCH ON ABUSE-DETERRENT OPIOIDS

It is time to engage in intelligent prognostication. There is plenty of reason for optimism.
- Lynn R. Webster, MD

As we have shown, opioids present considerable challenges when engaged as agents of abuse. However, opioids remain the most powerful analgesics and the only agents that provide relief for many conditions. As a result, there is a huge need to discover analgesics that retain their power yet are void of the significant adverse effects that can limit their effectiveness or cause harm. The search for the perfect analgesic is the Holy Grail of pain research.

The ideal opioid analgesic would not cause craving, would minimize withdrawal symptoms, and would not produce euphoria. This prototypical drug would deliver effective analgesia only for the duration of a pain event and would then dissipate, leaving behind no active metabolites. Such an opioid obviously does not yet exist.

In recent years, numerous sustained-release opioid formulations have been developed to provide better pain control via the continuous release of an active ingredient. Now, the focus of the pharmaceutical industry is turning toward the development of analgesics incorporating abuse deterrents that will improve safety and minimize adverse effects.

The Impetus for Opioid Research

Part of the pressure to produce safer medications comes from the FDA and the DEA, both of which are charged with protecting society. The stark alternative to the development of safer analgesics might be the government-enforced limitation of access to frequently abused medications. The drug market, driven by the needs of patients and the clinicians who treat them, is demanding better products that entail less risk of abuse, addiction, and diversion.

Education is only partially effective in curtailing drug abuse. One must accept that a community of "euphoria seekers" has been present throughout history and will not diminish. From John Keats to John Belushi, well-known personalities have abused consciousness-altering substances. Opiates are particularly prized among recreational drug users for the blissful psychogenic effects they produce, and no amount of "just saying no" will blunt the craving for drugs in some segments of society. The truly addicted are driven by a compulsion, divorced from any psychogenic reward, to consume drugs. Add to those realities the needs of patients with unrelieved pain or a mental disorder, and it is clear that admonishing people will never entirely prevent them from overusing their medications. Therefore, a leading research objective is to design formulations that remain effective as analgesics but prove less attractive to reward seekers. To accomplish this, drug developers seek to separate the beneficial pain-relieving properties of opioid analgesics from euphoric and other unwanted effects. The desired properties of an opioid include:

- Potent dose-related analgesia with no ceiling.
- Minimal adverse effects.
- Minimal abstinence syndrome.
- Minimal tolerance.
- No hyperalgesia.
- No euphoria.
- No stimulation of craving.

Areas of Abuse-Deterrent Research

In pursuit of abuse-deterrent opioids, most research is directed toward three general areas:

- The pharmacokinetics of opioid formulations.
- The pharmacodynamics of opioid analgesia.
- The pharmacogenetics of opioid analgesia.

Pharmacokinetics of Opioids

The term "pharmacokinetics" refers to the ways in which opioids are metabolized and distributed throughout the patient's system, including the rapidity of onset and the duration of action. The research in this area is concerned primarily with making it more difficult for a would-be abuser to extract an abusable portion of active pharmaceutical ingredient. Developing tamper-resistant formulations and adding aversive secondary ingredients to the current formulation are 2 major approaches. The goal is to limit the unintended release of the opioid from the formulation or to otherwise impede the inappropriate use of the drug.

Formulations That Release an Antagonist When Altered

One method of deterring inappropriate drug use is to introduce products in which tampering with the formulation releases an opioid antagonist that blocks or reverses the agonist effect. Tampering occurs because pleasure seekers constantly look for ways to increase the reward they get from abusing an opioid, particularly as tolerance to euphoria develops. Internet sites devoted to the support of recreational drug use are quick to report to other would-be abusers any successes experienced in circumventing barriers to abuse. These sites tell their readers how to extract an abusable portion of an active ingredient and how to alter formulations for alternate routes of administration. A main goal is to extract the opioid from the formulation so that it can be used at a higher-than-intended concentration. Known as "dose dumping," this can be accomplished in various ways.

One way to "dump" an opioid is to crush or grind the formulation, which causes more of the active ingredient to become available. The larger the opioid dose, the greater the amount of abusable ingredient released by this method. Another way of producing an enhanced effect is to dissolve the opioid formulation in water and then ingest or inject the solution. A third common method of dose dumping is to consume alcohol with the opioid. Alcohol can speed the rate of absorption and induce a premature release of active ingredient from some formulations. The FDA has increased its scrutiny of formulations that appear to be alcohol sensitive. This concern appears legitimate, because most unintentional overdose deaths occur in polysubstance users, and alcohol is a common substance found together with opioids after death.

To combat attempts at dose dumping, researchers are testing newer sustained-release opioid formulations that include an opioid antagonist, such as naltrexone, in addition to the therapeutic agonist agent. When taken as directed, the opioid is absorbed as intended with little or no absorption of the antagonist. However, crushing, damaging, or dissolving the drug; mixing it with alcohol; or otherwise manipulating the product will release the antagonist at doses sufficient to antagonize the opioid effects. Figure VIII:1 shows 2 examples of agonist-antagonist combinations. Capsule A consists of a naltrexone nucleus within an opioid matrix that releases the naltrexone only if the formulation is altered. Capsule B holds polymer-coated beads; some contain naltrexone and others contain an opioid. The beads look identical, but the opioid is released by the normal pH changes of the gastrointestinal tract; the thicker polymer coating of the naltrexone bead is not pH responsive and permits release of the agent only if the formulation is altered.

It is important to note that overuse of these drugs could still occur as patients seek more pain relief. Furthermore, adding an antagonist to the formulation could result in varying degrees of withdrawal, depending on the patient's tolerance to opioids and the amount of antagonist released when the product is altered. This approach could be considered a form of aversive therapy.

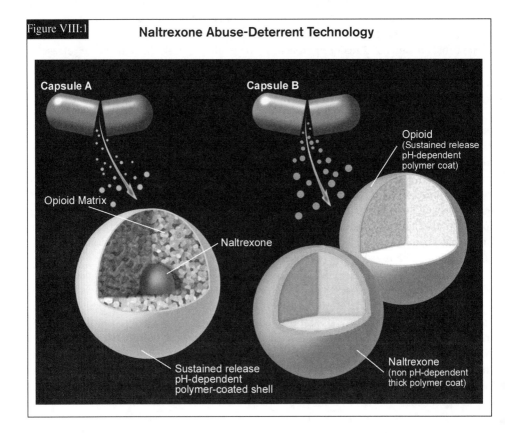

Figure VIII:1   **Naltrexone Abuse-Deterrent Technology**

What remains unclear is whether a dose of naltrexone can be a deterrent that prevents euphoria without blocking analgesia. Anecdotally, some patients with chronic pain who were treated in the first author's clinic for opioid addiction consistently reported the need for more opioid (to achieve a drug reward) than was necessary to provide pain relief. This suggests a potential therapeutic window during which an antagonist released from a formulation can lessen euphoria without reversing analgesia or inducing abstinence syndrome. Further research with abuse-deterrent formulations may help elucidate this potential relationship.

Gel Caps That Resist Crushing or Extraction

Several analgesic products purport to be time released, but most of the current time-release formulations appear susceptible to dose dumping. As a result, opioid researchers have produced several formulations designed to resist tampering. One is a gel cap that houses a sustained-release formula in a viscous base that is difficult to crush, freeze, heat, or dissolve in a liquid such as water or alcohol (Figure VIII:2). Oxycodone is the first opioid to be housed in this new gel capsule. Judging by its progress through clinical trials, this will be among the first abuse-resistant opioid agonist formulations to be introduced in the market.

Figure VIII:2	**Controlled-Release Gel Capsules Resist Alteration.**

Controlled-Release Gel Capsules Resist Alteration.
The viscous mass of oxycodone controlled release does not fracture. The controlled-release matrix is preserved.
Photo provided by Pain Therapeutics, Inc.

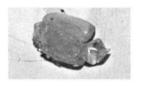

Simple laboratory tests can be used to simulate the common extraction techniques of crushing and stirring the medication into water or alcohol. Even grinding the gel capsule formulation in a coffee grinder could not yield enough oxycodone to be used in excess. One study[1] compared the pharmacokinetics of a controlled-release gel capsule containing oxycodone, an oxycodone controlled-release tablet, and an oxycodone immediate-release formula. Each of the 3 formulations was taken as intended, crushed in water, or crushed in alcohol. Some results of that experiment can be viewed in Figure VIII:3. Quantitative results from contrasting these formulations under all 3 conditions showed that the active pharmaceutical ingredient was markedly less extractable from the gel capsules than from commercial immediate- and sustained-release oxycodone tablets.[1] Swallowing the gel capsule whole produced oxycodone levels similar to those produced by conventional sustained-release formulas.

A major benefit of gel-cap technology is its imperviousness to the addition of alcohol. The spike in plasma levels after ingestion of the gel-cap formula that was crushed and dissolved in alcohol was less than half that observed from altering a conventional sustained-release formulation (Figure VIII:4). Tests using water showed similar tamper-resistant results: The gel-cap formulation yielded only a 20% release of oxycodone, and adding water to a conventional sustained-release formulation released 100% of the oxycodone (Figure VIII:5). However, people determined to abuse a formulation may still find ways to do so (perhaps by smoking the drug or by adulterant).

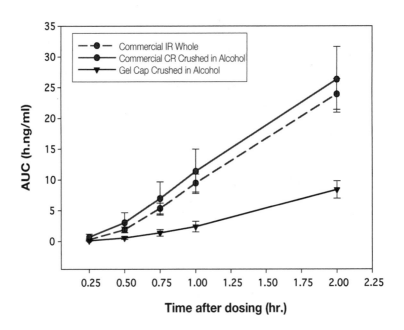

Figure VIII:3

Results of Head-to-Head Challenge Tests Comparing the Abuse Resistance of Capsules: Oxycodone Gel, Controlled Release, and Immediate Release

Gel Cap vs. Commercial CR:
Crushed & Taken with Alcohol

Legend:
- Commercial IR Whole
- Commercial CR Crushed in Alcohol
- Gel Cap Crushed in Alcohol

Y-axis: AUC (h.ng/ml)
X-axis: Time after dosing (hr.)

Source: Friedmann N, de Kater AW, Butera PG, Webster LR, Ratcliffe S, van Raders PA, Langford LM. Remoxy, a novel drug candidate, deters oxycodone abuse in humans [abstract]. 3rd International Congress World Institute of Pain, Barcelona, Spain; September 21-25 2004.

Formulas Containing an Added Irritant

A type of aversion therapy involves opioid formulations that are designed to release a noxious irritant if the drug is consumed recreationally. Capsaicin, the ingredient that gives chili peppers their heat, is one such irritant. When the drug is taken as directed, the capsaicin remains inactive. If the drug is chewed or crushed and is then snorted or injected, capsaicin acts as an agonist of the TRPV1 receptor (the receptor that contributes to heat-related pain). The result is an intense burning sensation that is extremely uncomfortable but causes no damage. Another similar invention combines an opioid with a sequestered emetic that would be released in sufficient quantity to cause vomiting if the product were altered. Such deterrents may be justified if they reduce the diversion of controlled substances for abuse.

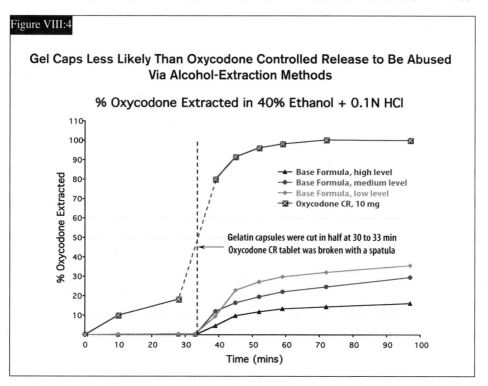

Figure VIII:4

Gel Caps Less Likely Than Oxycodone Controlled Release to Be Abused Via Alcohol-Extraction Methods

% Oxycodone Extracted in 40% Ethanol + 0.1N HCl

Legend:
- Base Formula, high level
- Base Formula, medium level
- Base Formula, low level
- Oxycodone CR, 10 mg

Gelatin capsules were cut in half at 30 to 33 min
Oxycodone CR tablet was broken with a spatula

y-axis: % Oxycodone Extracted
x-axis: Time (mins)

Pharmacodynamics of Opioids

The term "pharmacodynamics" refers to the action of drugs on specific opioid receptors. In general, the pharmacodynamic response depends on the receptor to which the substance binds, the affinity of the substance for the receptor, and whether the substance is an agonist or an antagonist. Some opioid receptors produce more analgesia, and others produce respiratory depression, dysphoria, etc.

Research on Opioid Receptors

A focus of research on opioids is to develop ligands that bind to opioid receptors to preferentially stimulate the desired effect of analgesia while preventing unwanted effects such as euphoria, tolerance, physical dependence, or the heightened pain response of hyperalgesia. It appears that most of the analgesic action of opioids (in addition to many adverse effects such as euphoria) occurs at the mu-opioid receptors. Most clinically delivered opioids are mu agonists, and most research has centered on manipulating mu-opioid receptors and their subtypes. However, because opioids do not bind to just 1 type of receptor, this presents both challenges and opportunities for opioid researchers.

Delta and kappa receptors have presented problems for opioid researchers in the past. Delta agonists are ineffective against pain and may cause convulsions, and centrally acting kappa agonists produce dysphoria. Today, however, more recent research into peripheral kappa receptors is showing some promise in the amelioration of pain conditions such as hyperalgesia.[2] Delta antagonists may also be of value in preventing opioid tolerance. Al-

---

Figure VIII:5

Gel Caps Less Likely to Be Abused Via Water-Extraction Methods

Oxycodone controlled-release gel capsule after being frozen, crushed, and ground with water (as shown on left). Oxycodone controlled-release tablet after being crushed and ground with water (as shown on right).

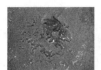

Oxycodone extracted: 20%   Oxycodone extracted: 100%

---

though conclusions have not yet been established, a greater understanding of complex neuromodulatory systems may enable more selective targeting of sites by pharmaceuticals to produce desired benefits.

Reducing Drug Reward

Continued drug abuse rewires the nervous system. The systemic changes induced by drug abuse are profound. If scientists can better understand the cellular and molecular details of that altered circuitry, effective treatments for addiction that target the underlying compulsion could be developed. A promising approach to safer opioid analgesia is to reduce the drug reward valued by abusers. This task is complex because the neuromodulatory system that establishes and perpetuates drug reward is influenced by interdependent factors.

One potential research target is the formation of drug-related memories that drive repeated behavior. Scientists are now experimenting with ways to essentially erase the memory of drug abuse. The place preference demonstrated by addicted rats, which associate their desired substance with a particular chamber of the cage, is of interest to scientists in that regard. Laboratory tests have achieved some success in disrupting the transference of place preference to long-term memory by injecting substances that alter the protein synthesis process of the brain.[3] The rats studied simply stopped associating the place at which they received their drug reward with the agent they wanted to obtain. The practical benefits of and ethical concerns associated with the use of such a technology in humans are unknown.

Mice that lack various G-protein–coupled receptors and their ligands demonstrate diminished drug reward.[4] Preliminary work suggests that some addictive substances do not directly activate mu receptors but depend on the release of certain opioid peptides that then activate mu receptors. If an intact endogenous opioid system is needed to establish drug reward, blocking the pathways involved could reduce the reward not only from opioids but from other addictive behaviors involving food, strenuous exercise, tetrahydrocannabinol, and nicotine. Research also has implicated cannabinoid-1 (CB-1), substance P and neurokinin 1 (NK-1) receptors in drug reward. Laboratory mice lacking NK-1 or CB-1 receptors appear to receive analgesia but no reward from morphine.[4] This is an exciting discovery because of its potential therapeutic value. CB-1 antagonists may represent a new generation of compounds that could be used to treat drug addiction and could be combined with opioid agonists to reduce abuse during pain therapy. Possibilities such as these suggest a neurobiologic pathway that could be exploited via the body's endogenous reward system to reduce the euphoric impact of clinical opioids. Much depends on isolating and targeting the appropriate receptors and subtypes.

The reducing of reward and the lessening of tolerance, physical dependence, and hyperalgesia should theoretically significantly reduce drug-seeking aberrant behavior in chronic-pain patients. This is likely to be true for most such patients. However, the end result of a reduction in drug reward for a person with the disease of addiction is less clear. In some animal models, the reduction of drug reward only made the animal work harder to obtain the desired drug. It is important to remember that the disease of addiction is marked by compulsive consumption that is independent of any reward and that persists even in the presence of adverse consequences.

The Promise of Peripheral Action

A driving theory behind opioid research posits that central nervous system access is required to stimulate the drug reward center. It follows logically that opioid formulations that spare the central nervous system while producing strong analgesic effects on peripheral systems could have great potential for decreasing drug reward. By blocking access to the central nervous system, the body's reward center could be spared stimulation.

It is clear that peripheral opioid receptors mediate analgesia, but it is not known how much analgesia can be produced with only peripheral opioid receptor stimulation. The local administration of opiates at the site of injury results in sufficient analgesia that appears to be augmented by a preexisting inflammation. In fact, tissue damage has been shown to enhance analgesia by stimulating opioid receptors at the periphery, perhaps by enhancing G-protein coupling.[5] Uninjured nerves do not produce the same increased response to opioids.

In animal models, peripheral opioids have been shown to be effective in the treatment of several types of typically opioid-resistant pain, including neuropathic pain.[5] If the research goal can be achieved, peripheral opioids could be safer, more precise, and less likely to induce abuse than are centrally acting opioids. This type of targeted pain relief offers great promise for the future.

Preventing Heightened Pain Sensitivity

Opioid withdrawal is known to precipitate hyperalgesia, which is an increased sensitivity to pain. Even in the absence of withdrawal, heightened pain sensitivity (which is indicated by a lowered pain threshold) can occur after long-term opioid administration.[6] Opioid-induced hyperalgesia has been observed in both animal and human experimental models.[7]

Current theories suggest that excitatory amino acid receptors, such as the N-methyl-D-aspartate (NMDA) receptor, influence the development of opioid-induced hyperalgesia and tolerance.[6] NMDA receptors also appear to play a critical role in the development of central sensitization, which is a complicated mechanism of increased pain sensitivity.[8] Central sensitization precipitates actual changes in cellular structure and function. The clinical implications are that the use of an NMDA antagonist could slow the development of tolerance and prevent or even reverse the progress of abnormal pain sensitivity.[8] The value for abuse deterrence lies in the removal of an incentive to overuse pain medication. However, early investigational research has shown that centrally acting NMDA antagonists could produce central nervous system toxicity. As a result, research in that area is limited.

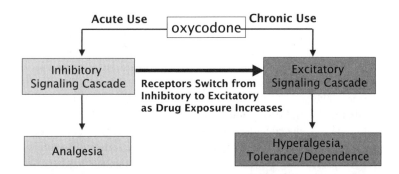

Figure VIII:6a

Opioid Hyperalgesia, Tolerance, and Dependence Stem from a Switch in Signaling

Inhibitory ⟶ Excitatory

Opioid Tolerance/Dependence is a Switch in Signaling

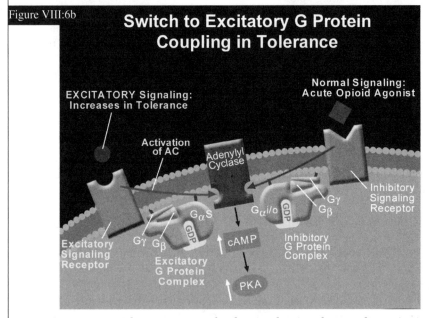

Figure VIII:6b

Switch to Excitatory G Protein Coupling in Tolerance

Long-term opioid exposure may lead to analgesic tolerance by excitation of the adenylyl cyclase-cAMP pathway. A switch in G-protein coupling by opioid receptors from Gi/o to Gs activates adenylyl cyclase and interferes with the G (beta gamma) inhibition of voltage-dependent calcium channels. Coadministration of an ultra–low-dose opioid antagonist blocks the G-protein uncoupling and delays or may reverse opioid-associated tolerance and dependence.

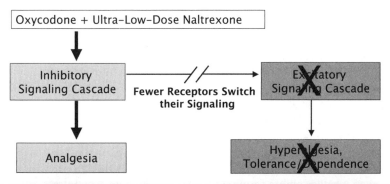

Figure VIII:7a

Cotreatment with an Ultra–Low-Dose Antagonist Prevents Excitatory Signaling

Inhibitory —/↛ Excitatory

Ultra–Low–Dose Antagonist Prevents Excitatory Signaling

Oxycodone + Ultra–Low–Dose Naltrexone

| Inhibitory Signaling Cascade | Fewer Receptors Switch their Signaling | Excitatory Signaling Cascade |

Analgesia

Hyperalgesia, Tolerance/Dependence

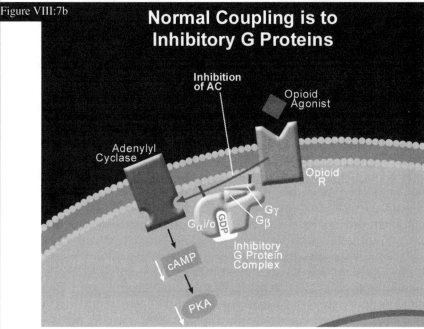

Figure VIII:7b

Normal Coupling is to Inhibitory G Proteins

Inhibition of AC

Opioid Agonist

Adenylyl Cyclase

Opioid R

Gγ
Gβ

G$_{\alpha i/o}$ GDP

Inhibitory G Protein Complex

cAMP

PKA

Acute opioid administration activates the mu-opioid receptor-linked inhibitory G-protein. The adenylyl cyclase-cAMP pathway is inhibited by activation of the inhibitory proteins. The G (beta gamma) dimer is released from the Gi/o complex. This leads to inhibition of both voltage-dependent calcium channels and cellular activity and results in analgesia.

Opioids and Ultra–Low-Dose Antagonists

As noted in the section titled "Pharmacokinetics," adding an antagonist to an opioid formulation may help to deter dose dumping. An antagonist performs another function as well: At an ultra-low dose it can act as a receptor modulator. Early test data indicate that a formula containing a minuscule amount of opioid antagonist in combination with an opioid agonist may block some of the drug-related reward, slow the buildup of tolerance and physical dependence, and extend the action of analgesia.[9] In addition, there is evidence of a lower incidence of abstinence syndrome when the drug is stopped. These are attractive clinical benefits.

Early evidence indicates that ultra–low-dose antagonist cotreatment derives some of its efficacy from the restoration of normal G-protein coupling patterns. After long-term opioid treatment, opioid receptors begin to adapt to the continuous-stimulation agonist. The result is an uncoupling of the G-protein, which leads to excitatory signaling rather than the usual inhibitory signaling (Figures VIII:6a and VIII:6b). The mechanism of action switches from normal Gi/Go coupling to Gs coupling. In this way, the excitatory effects of opioids appear to contribute to opioid tolerance, hyperalgesia, and physical dependence.[10-11] If 1 ng of antagonist is added to the formulation, fewer receptors switch their coupling, and this slows the development of tolerance and other adverse effects caused by treatment with an opioid (Figures VIII:7a and VIII:7b).

However, whether opioid formulations that incorporate even ultra-low doses of antagonist can provide sufficient pain relief for patients with the worst types of chronic pain has not been determined. In a Phase II study of patients with moderate-to-severe osteoarthritis, an oxycodone-naltrexone combination administered twice a day produced significantly greater pain relief than did placebo, oxycodone administered 4 times daily, or the same oxycodone-naltrexone combination administered 4 times daily.[12] It is notable that the subjects who received the agonist-antagonist combination twice daily received less antagonist than did patients who received 4 doses daily; therefore, the amount of naltrexone included in the daily dose seems to be an important factor.

In a Phase III trial of 719 patients with severe chronic low-back pain, those treated with a combination of oxycodone and ultra–low-dose naltrexone reported pain relief comparable to that provided by oxycodone alone.[9] Those in the oxycodone-naltrexone group also reported 50% fewer symptoms of physical dependence and withdrawal than did patients treated with oxycodone. Overall, the oxycodone-naltrexone group experienced 20% fewer opioid-related adverse effects (including somnolence, pruritus, and moderate-to-severe constipation) during treatment than did patients treated with oxycodone. Of particular note was the finding of less physical dependence when naltrexone was added to oxycodone. It is true that physical dependence is distinct from addiction and is a predictable physiologic result of long-term opioid therapy. However, patients and physicians sometimes associate physical dependence on drugs strictly with addiction and either reduce opioid therapy or forego it altogether, even when it is needed for pain control. Also, many patients as well as recreational drug users become "hooked" on painkilling drugs because their fear of withdrawal symptoms makes it nearly impossible to discontinue drug use. In short, pain relief without physical dependence is a most desirable clinical benefit. With that in mind, it should be understood that opioid formulations that use ultra-low doses of antagonist only slow (but do not prevent) the development of tolerance and physical dependence.

Pharmacogenetics

Research into the genetics of pain and addiction could lead to pharmacologic advances that would help to prevent abuse by patients treated with an opioid. Gaining a better understanding of the great genetic variability in opioid response among individuals could help to identify those most likely to experience benefit or harm from opioid therapy. This area of research opens the door to the design of opioids that are less likely to stimulate the reward center and that exert more extensive effects on the opioid receptor subunits that induce analgesia. In the future, prescribing the right drug may depend on the genotype of the individual, and it may be possible to determine from the patient's genetic profile which drugs will deliver the best analgesia and prevent abuse.

The mapping of the human genome offers immense opportunities for pain researchers. Although the expense of this type of clinical application is still prohibitive in most instances, the cost of genotyping likely will decrease rapidly in coming years. A systematic research approach could uncover much data valuable to the invention of new pain-relief technologies. Genetic therapies require greater sophistication than medical science now possesses, but the future of opioid genetic research appears virtually limitless.

Individual Genetic Variations

Physicians who treat pain have long known that the response to opioids varies widely among individuals. Differences in the bioavailability of the drug and the patient's response to pain stimuli explain some (but not all) of that difference. The genetic makeup of individual patients is likely a strong factor. This theory is supported by known variations among ethnic groups in response to opioid medications. When treated with an opioid, whites become more sedated and exhibit more respiratory depression than do Asians; Native Americans display even more depression of the ventilatory response than do whites.[13-14] The theory is bolstered further by evidence that inbred laboratory mice (CXBK) show no response to levels of morphine that are analgesic for more than 90% of typical mice.[15]

Additional laboratory observations supporting genetic variation as a factor in opioid response include the following findings:

- A polymorphism of the MDR1 gene may determine the toxic effects of morphine.
- A deoxyribonucleic acid sequence variance in the CYP2D6 gene prevents the metabolic change of codeine to morphine, altering codeine's analgesic properties.
- Polymorphisms at the mu-opioid receptors and sex differences appear to influence variable responses to opioids.[16]

Variations in the amino acid sequence and its potential effect on the efficacy of opioids is an area ripe for further research and is likely only the tip of a very large iceberg of genetic complexity. It has already been shown that a variation in amino acid sequence at the mu receptor can change receptor signaling after stimulation with morphine.[17]

There is new information, too, about the role that the mu receptor may play in the disease of addiction. Approximately 30 genes that contribute to or mediate the properties of

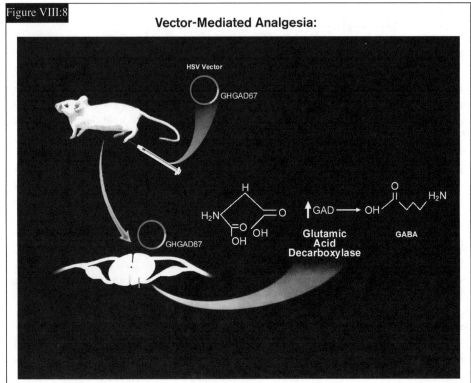

In a murine model, the injection of nonreplicating herpes simplex virus (HSV) vector containing GHGAD67 coding for glutamic acid decarboxylase (GAD) is used to transduce the dorsal root ganglion to produce GAD. This increased production of GAD at the dorsal horn ganglion converts glutamic acid to gamma-amino butyric acid (GABA). GABA is an inhibitory neurotransmitter that blocks the transmission of an impulse from 1 cell to another in the central nervous system, thus preventing the overfiring of nerve cells. This vector-mediated gene transfer has been shown to reduce chronic neuropathic pain caused by lumbar root injury in rodents.

addiction have been identified. Targeting either the gene or the modifiers of gene expression may lead to new analgesics that are less likely to cause addiction.

Differences in the ways in which people manifest pain are also probably influenced by genetics. Research[18] with inbred mice indicates variations in behavioral responses to more than 20 different pain conditions, which suggests a genetic basis underlying pain processing. However, familial inheritance of pain syndromes has not been observed or documented thus far.[18] Allele-based association studies may someday shed light on the mystery of why pain persists in some patients but not others after nearly identical tissue damage.

At present, nearly 200 candidate genes that may be involved in pain processing have been identified,[18] and there may be thousands more. Studies of pain candidate genes may help to determine which of hundreds of potential analgesic targets are worthy of further attention, and the development of novel medications may result. A diagnostic test for the risk of chronic pain is not out of the question. Genetic studies could even illuminate the links between chronic pain and the frequent codiagnoses of depression, anxiety, and substance abuse. These are exciting avenues of research.

Gene Transfer Technology

Another intriguing area of research involves gene transfer therapy. This is a process of stimulating opioid production at sites of injury while bypassing central adverse effects. Scientists are working on ways of delivering genes containing pain-suppressing drugs or other products to damaged nerve cells to block the transmission of pain signals from the nerves to the brain. Research combining peripheral opioids with gene therapy suggests that opioid-producing immune cells can be sent to damaged tissues to secrete opioids.[5] Also, sensory neurons at peripheral sites produce opioid peptides, which may be stimulated to overexpress through gene transfer therapy.[5]

One avenue of research involves transferring the gene coding for glutamic acid decarboxylase (GAD) and delivering it to nerve cells in the dorsal root ganglion near the spine by means of a vector or disabled virus (Figure VIII:8). An enzyme generated by GAD triggers the release of GABA, the powerful neurotransmitter known to block pain signals and the absence of which is linked to the development of neuropathic pain. The pain-suppressing effect of this therapy lasted up to 6 weeks in laboratory rats.[19] Direct delivery to the focal site within the nervous system can eliminate the sedating effect that has thus far limited the feasibility of GABA-centered treatments. Research such as this is still years away from producing useful clinical interventions for patients, but early results suggest that progress is being made toward more carefully targeted and less harmful treatments for pain.

Paradigm Shifts

Matching Analgesia to Physiology

The abuse of opioids may be influenced as much by their manner of use as by their own intrinsic euphorigenic properties. It is clear that the undertreatment of pain can lead to aberrant behavior. However, it is also possible that not synchronizing opioid therapy to the body's normal circadian rhythms may also lead to aberrant behavior. Perhaps it is wise to reexamine the broadly accepted conventional paradigms pertaining to opioid prescribing.

Current best practice in the management of chronic intractable nonmalignant pain usually calls for the administration of a sustained-release (12-hour or 24-hour) opioid to relieve persistent pain plus a short-acting agent to combat episodes of breakthrough pain. However, when opioids are prescribed around the clock, some patients experience hypofunctioning of the endocrine and immune systems. The result is a lowered pain threshold and an increased demand for analgesics. If opioid blood levels could mimic the circadian rhythm, the impact on the endocrine and immune systems might be lessened and pain control enhanced. This theory, of course, is only speculative at this time, but studies are under way to examine that concept.

Is There a Ceiling Dose of Opioids?

During the past 2 decades, research in pain control has revealed that much higher doses of opioids can be prescribed for chronic nonmalignant pain than were previously believed to be safe or advisable. Will the future involve a change in that view? Do higher doses of opioids lead to drug abuse or addiction after all? Pain physicians resist establishing an arbitrary ceiling for opioid prescribing, and rightly so. Patients are so individual in their responses to medication that an effective analgesic dose in 1 patient could be toxic or lethal in another. Pain treatment, like all medicine, must be individualized to be effective. However, a belief that opioid tolerance protects a patient from the serious adverse effects of opioid use may foster a false sense of security in some pain physicians. It is true that very high doses can be safely administered in chronic-pain patients who are opioid tolerant. Does that mean, however, that the sky is the limit? Is there absolute protection? Of course not. Judicious use of opioids with vigilant management is mandatory.

The *New England Journal of Medicine* waded into this unresolved debate with an article suggesting that limits on opioid dosing may be needed.[20] Although many pain specialists decided that the authors' assertion (ie, that daily opioid doses of higher than 180 mg could be excessive for chronic-pain patients) was alarmist, the larger point of the article was often missed. The authors were not attempting to set a nonbreachable ceiling dose for all chronic-pain patients but were pointing out the dearth of research demonstrating the efficacy and safety of higher doses of opioids. That is a point well worth considering. Optimal pain relief is not always achieved by unrestricted escalation of the dosage of an opioid. Furthermore, any opioids prescribed in excess of medical need could be made available for illegal sale or abuse.

These thoughts do not mean that clinicians should fear prescribing adequate medication or fail to titrate dosages to an optimal analgesic level. To accomplish that, many considerations come into play. The ceiling dose of 1 drug may not equal that of another. The factors affecting an adequate dosage include the patient's pain level, general health, concomitant medications, age, sex, type of pain, experience with opioids, and the presence of complicating conditions such as heart disease or sleep apnea. In an opioid-tolerant patient with chronic intractable pain and no other drug treatment, 240 mg per day of oxycodone might not be too much medication. A patient with a similar pain condition who is also taking benzodiazepines for anxiety might need to cut the opioid dosage in half.

The authors of the article in *New England Journal of Medicine* cited above summarize the matter thus:

"… attempts to limit the escalation of the opioid dose sometimes fail. If dose escalation is unsuccessful, it is crucial to ask whether the opioid used is effective in treating the patient's chronic pain."[20]

Conclusion

Euphoria is an opioid effect sought by patients who want to abuse drugs prescribed for pain. The first objective of opioid research is to find methods of reducing the euphoria, tolerance, hyperalgesia, and other undesired effects of opioids while retaining their analgesic properties. Failure to confront the problems presented by the adverse effects of opioid treatment will risk a reduction in their availability for use in legitimate medical practice. The ability to provide better pain relief with fewer adverse effects would reduce the consequences of drug misuse, which is our primary goal.

Judging from the current research, the future holds a cornucopia of choices for the treatment of chronic pain. For at least the next decade, however, and probably beyond, opioids will continue to constitute the mainstay of pain control. Clinicians can benefit patients by continuing to learn about the new developments in pain management and addiction control and by continuing their commitment to the safe and effective administration of opioids.

References

1. Friedman N, de Kater A, Butera PG, Webster LR, Ratcliffe S, Langford RM. Remoxy, a novel drug candidate deters oxycodone abuse in humans [Abstract]. Pain Med. 2005; 6(2):180-181.
2. Coop A, MacKerell AD Jr. The future of opioid analgesics. Am J Pharm Educ. 2003; 66:153-156.
3. Miller CA, Marshall JF. Molecular substrates for retrieval and reconsolidation of cocaine-associated contextual memory. Neuron. 2005 Sep 15;47(6):873-84.
4. Bryant CD, Zaki PA, Carroll FI, Evans CJ. Opioids and addiction: Emerging pharmaceutical strategies for reducing reward and opponent processes. Clin Neurosci Res. 2005;5:103-15.
5. Stein C, Schafer M, Machelska H. Attacking pain at its source: new perspectives on opioids. Nat Med. 2003 Aug;9(8):1003-8.
6. Mao J. Opioid-induced abnormal pain sensitivity: implications in clinical opioid therapy. Pain. 2002 Dec;100(3):213-7.
7. Koppert W. [Opioid-induced analgesia and hyperalgesia]. Schmerz. 2005 Oct;19(5):386-90, 392-4. German.
8. Simonnet G. [Complexity and physiology of the analgesic effects of opioids]. Rev Med Suisse 2005 Jun 22;1(25):1682-5.
9. Webster LR, Butera PG, Moran LV, Wu N, Burns LH, Friedmann N. Oxytrex minimizes physical dependence while providing effective analgesia: a randomized controlled trial in low back pain. J Pain. 2006 Dec;7(12):937-46.
10. Wang HY, Friedman E, Olmstead MC, Burns LH. Ultra-low-dose naloxone suppresses opioid tolerance, dependence and associated changes in mu opioid receptor-G protein coupling and Gbetagamma signaling. Neuroscience. 2005;135(1):247-61.
11. Crain SM, Shen KF. Antagonists of excitatory opioid receptor functions enhance morphine's analgesic potency and attenuate opioid tolerance/dependence liability. Pain. 2000 Feb;84(2-3):121-31.
12. Chindalore VL, Craven RA, Yu KP, Butera PG, Burns LH, Friedmann N. Adding ultralow-dose naltrexone to oxycodone enhances and prolongs analgesia: a randomized, controlled trial of Oxytrex. J Pain. 2005 Jun;6(6):392-9.
13. Zhou HH, Sheller JR, Nu H, Wood M, Wood AJ. Ethnic differences in response to morphine. Clin Pharmacol Ther. 1993 Nov;54(5):507-13.
14. Cepeda MS, Farrar JT, Roa JH, Boston R, Meng QC, Ruiz F, Carr DB, Strom BL. Ethnicity influences morphine pharmacokinetics and pharmacodynamics. Clin Pharmacol Ther. 2001 Oct;70(4):351-61.
15. Schuller AG, King MA, Zhang J, Bolan E, Pan YX, Morgan DJ, Chang A, Czick ME, Unterwald EM, Pasternak GW, Pintar JE. Retention of heroin and morphine-6 beta-glucuronide analgesia in a new line of mice lacking exon 1 of MOR-1. Nat Neurosci. 1999 Feb;2(2):151-6.

16. Foley KM. Opioids and chronic neuropathic pain. N Engl J Med 2003 Mar 27;348(13):1279-81.
17. Befort K, Filliol D, Decaillot FM, Gaveriaux-Ruff C, Hoehe MR, Kieffer BL. A single nucleotide polymorphic mutation in the human mu-opioid receptor severely impairs receptor signaling. J Biol Chem. 2001 Feb 2;276(5):3130-7. Epub 2000 Nov 6.
18. Belfer I, Wu T, Kingman A, Krishnaraju RK, Goldman D, Max MB. Candidate gene studies of human pain mechanisms: methods for optimizing choice of polymorphisms and sample size. Anesthesiology. 2004 Jun;100(6):1562-72.
19. Hao S, Mata M, Wolfe D, Huang S, Glorioso JC, Fink DJ. Gene transfer of glutamic acid decarboxylase reduces neuropathic pain. Ann Neurol. 2005 Jun;57(6):914-8. Erratum in: Ann Neurol. 2005 Nov;58(5):818. Huang, Shaohua [added].
20. Ballantyne JC, Mao J. Opioid therapy for chronic pain. N Engl J Med. 2003 Nov 13;349(20):1943-53.

SUMMARY

The first known written mention of the poppy plant, from which opium derives, appears in a Sumerian text from the 4th century BC.[1] Early healers hailed it as a "plant of joy." Even centuries later, some physicians believed that this agony-relieving substance arose from a divine origin. The heavenly properties of opium, however, did not come risk free.

Today, some scientists and medical professionals characterize the treatment of pain with pharmaceutical opiates as an anachronism or an "embarrassment that should go the way of leeches."[2] Although opiates are an ancient treatment for pain, they still provide an effective and even life-saving therapy for many patients. As analgesics, opioids are peerless. They reduce most types of pain by at least 30% percent, on average.[3] Research indicates that when opioid treatment for chronic pain is stopped suddenly, patients experience more pain and a reduced quality of life — not an uncontrolled craving for drugs.[4] Few medications boast such an efficacious profile. Results like these matter even more now, when serious questions are being raised about the increased potential for heart attack and stroke associated with cyclooxygenase-2 inhibitors.

However, opioids are not a panacea. *Time Magazine* reports that approximately half of all US chronic-pain patients simply do not find a good analgesic solution.[5] It is also true that a substantial number of individuals treated for addiction to an opioid or another substance will experience a recurrence of addiction that will be permanent in some cases. These are difficult realities. However, they do not mean that treatment is futile. No other disease boasts a cure rate of 100%, and no other treatment regimen commands total patient compliance with medical direction. Neither should the fields of pain and addiction medicine be subject to unworkable expectations.

Finding the right professional for the job is the first priority. Patients should question their family doctors on attitudes toward pain treatment and, when appropriate, should seek referrals. Healthcare providers should consult with specialists in a variety of related fields when indicated to ensure that patients find and receive the best treatment available. Pain treatment is not synonymous with the prescribing of opioids, and a number of very effective nonpharmacologic options are available. The National Pain Foundation provides information on clinical options on its Web site.[6] However, if opioids are indeed best, clinicians should not allow misguided fears to interfere with effective therapy.

Although many questions remain unanswered, most people who take medications for pain will not become addicted to them, and most abuse problems can be managed. These conclusions should never be taken for granted, however. All clinicians who prescribe opioids should remain vigilant. They must screen patients for the possibility of drug abuse and clearly outline the goals of treatment before therapy is initiated. They should also continue to monitor patients, understand all regulations that apply to the use of opioids, and look to the future, when opioid prescribing will become a safer, more exact science.

References

1. Booth M. *Opium: A History*. 1st US ed.. New York, NY: Thomas Dunne Books; 1998.
2. Stix G. A toxin against pain. Sci Am. 2005 Apr;292(4):70-5.
3. Kalso E, Edwards JE, Moore RA, McQuay HJ. Opioids in chronic non-cancer pain: systematic review of efficacy and safety. Pain. 2004 Dec;112(3):372-80. Review.
4. Cowan DT, Wilson-Barnett J, Griffiths P, Vaughan DJ, Gondhia A, Allan LG. A randomized, double-blind, placebo-controlled, cross-over pilot study to assess the effects of long-term opioid drug consumption and subsequent abstinence in chronic non-cancer pain patients receiving controlled-release morphine. Pain Med. 2005 Mar-Apr;6(2):113-21.
5. Wallis C. The right (and wrong) way to treat pain. Time Magazine. 2005; February 20.
6. My treatment: treatment options. National Pain Foundation. Available at: http://www.NationalPainFoundation.org. Accessed April 10, 2007.